D1156877

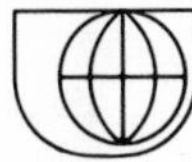

World University Library

The World University Library is an international series of books, each of which has been specially commissioned. The authors are leading scientists and scholars from all over the world who, in an age of increasing specialisation, see the need for a broad, up-to-date presentation of their subject. The aim is to provide authoritative introductory books for students which will be of interest also to the general reader. Publication of the series takes place in Britain, France, Germany, Holland, Italy, Spain, Sweden and the United States.

P. Lain Entralgo

Doctor and Patient

translated from the Spanish
by Frances Partridge

World University Library

McGraw-Hill Book Company
New York Toronto

Library of Congress Catalog Card Number: 68-21841
Phototypeset by BAS Printers Limited, Wallop, Hampshire, England
Printed by Officine Grafiche Arnoldo Mondadori, Verona, Italy

Contents

Why is it that I owe something more to my physician and my teacher, and yet do not complete the payment of what is due to them? Because from being physician and teacher they become friends, and we are under an obligation to them, not because of their skill, which they sell, but because of their kind and friendly goodwill.

If, therefore, a physician does nothing more than feel my pulse and put me on the list of those whom he visits on his rounds, instructing me what to do and what to avoid without any personal feeling, I owe him nothing more than his fee, because he does not see me as a friend but as a client . . .

Why then, are we so much indebted to these men? Not because what they have sold us is worth more than we paid for it, but because they have contributed something to us personally. A physician who gave me more attention than was necessary, because he was afraid for me, not for his professional reputation, who was not content to indicate remedies, but also applied them; who sat at my bedside among my anxious friends, and hurried to me at times of crisis; for whom no service was too burdensome, none too distasteful to perform; who was not indifferent to my moans; to whom, although a host of others sent for him, I was always his chief concern; who took time for the others only when my illness permitted him.

Such a man has placed me under an obligation, not so much as a physician but as a friend.

Seneca, *de Beneficiis,* VI, 16

Introduction

Until well into this century, it was only very rarely that the relationship between doctor and patient presented problems, when the doctor failed to observe the rules, or when the patient for one reason or another lost confidence in the man who was attending him. But during the last few decades the situation appears to have changed entirely, and there now seems some degree of conflict present even in a normal relationship between the patient and doctor.

There are several reasons for this change, the following among them. In the first place, the great technical developments in diagnosis and treatment – radiography, chemical analysis, electrography – often now prevent a sufficiently 'human' contact being established. In other cases, the practice of psychotherapy – or, more simply, a therapeutic relationship with the 'persona' of the invalid – produces the phenomena of the transference, in the psychoanalytical sense of the word, and these phenomena invariably give rise to conflict. Thirdly, the increasing socialisation of medical care, and its resulting mass-production, often depersonalise the relationship, by emphasising its contractual character and limiting the time the doctor can devote to the patient to a disturbing and harmful extent. Finally, enlightened by the resources of so-called 'mass-culture' – including a great many advertisements of pharmaceutical products – the patient usually takes a hand in his own treatment, often in opposition to his doctor.

As a result of all these factors, the doctor-patient relationship has become less natural, so to speak, than for centuries it was, or appeared to be; and this has shown how vital it is to the proper practice of medicine. Accurate diagnosis and correct choice of therapeutic measures are necessary conditions for good treatment, but they are not the only ones. Good treatment also depends on a satisfactory relation between the invalid and his doctor – the first of all remedies, as Balint describes it.

I propose to examine, historically and systematically, what this relation was like in the past, what it is now, and what I think it ought to be. But before beginning, I think it would be desirable to give a brief synopsis of the nature and basic structure of a medical 'event'. By this I mean every technical contact between doctor and patient, whether diagnostic or therapeutic in character. It seems to me that its nature and structure can be summed up in the following points:

1 Generically speaking, a medical event is a *meeting* between two men, such that its content, form and development are controlled by the conscious and unconscious intentions of both at the moment of meeting. If their relationship is to be satisfactory it is essential that the doctor's chief purpose should be to give technical help, and the patient's to get well; but, as we shall see, this is not always the case.

2 A genuine mutual link between the intentions of the doctor and patient constitutes the *basis* of the medical event, and upon this are constructed the four main factors expressing it and giving it reality: (a) the *cognitive aspect*, technically described as 'diagnosis'; (b) the *operative aspect*, usually known as 'treatment'; (c) the *affective aspect*, understood as 'friendship' by the ancient Greeks, or as 'transference' by modern psychoanalysts; and (d) the *ethico-religious aspect*,

given shape in each case by the customs and beliefs current in the world to which doctor and patient belong.

3 A medical event is both *personal* and *social* in character. It is personal in that it happens between two people. It is social in that patient and doctor exist within a society which to a very large extent conditions their way of life and the manner of their meeting. Unless this twofold character is taken into account, the relation between doctor and patient cannot be properly understood.

Let us now see how this scheme corresponds with historical facts, and with what is happening at the present day.

Part 1:
The doctor-patient relationship in history

1 Classical Greece

Before the days of Alcmaeon of Croton and Hippocrates in the fifth century BC, medicine in ancient Greece was, as in the rest of the world, a combination of empiricism and magic, given a Hellenic pattern. The military surgeons of the *Iliad* and the sedentary or itinerant healers – periodeutics and rhizotomists – of pre-Hippocratic medicine, were more or less skilful empirics; while the other methods of healing in force – such as incubation in the temples of Asclepius, magic spells and cathartic rites – revealed the magic mentality just as clearly. So it went on until the fifth century BC.

All through that century, for reasons that are now unimportant, men from the Greek colonial cities – such as Croton, Agrigentum, Cos, Cnidus – were inventing a new approach to the care of the sick. Empiric medicine had consisted in repeating any treatment that had been found beneficial in any individual case, while magic claimed to manipulate powerful superhuman forces by means of special rituals. Resolutely abandoning both, the new technique – known as *technê iatrikê*, or 'the art of healing' when applied to medicine – consisted in acting with some degree of scientifically exact knowledge of *what* was being done, and *why*. Technique, in fact, is the knowledge how to act according to the *what* and the *why*.

With Alcmaeon of Croton and Hippocrates, and ever since their time, a 'technical' doctor has needed three sorts of knowledge: he must know what the illness is (which involves knowing something about his patient as a man); what is the remedy that will cure it; and why that remedy acts as a cure in such a disease but not in others. From the intellectual basis of *physiologia* (or natural science in general) which had been elaborated a little earlier by the pre-Socratic philosophers – Pythagoras, Empedocles and Democritus in particular – sprang the sciences of human *physiologia* (anatomy and physiology, in modern terminology), *pharmakologia* or natural science of medicines, *pathologia* or natural science of the forms of disease, and *technê therapeutikê* or scientific doctrine of treatment. In opposition to the 'empiric', the magician, the exorcist and the priest of Asclepius – but without completely replacing them – technical followers of Asclepius, or Asclepiads, now began to practise, and medicine was ever afterwards to be understood as the art of healing, as the various writings of the *Corpus Hippocraticum* defined it.

Does this mean that, within the framework of this technical view of medicine, the relationship between doctor and patient in ancient Greece was a uniform one? This is what most historical studies of the subject lead one to suppose; but a careful examination of the sources – in this case the dialogues of Plato – reveals a very different state of things, for this relation varied greatly according to whether the sick man were a rich freeman, a poor freeman, or a slave. With this reservation, I will begin by setting forth what may be considered as the canon of Greek medicine when the protagonists were an educated patient and an Asclepiad.

The concept of philia

Let us imagine a typical medical event. Apart from his economic and professional interests, the doctor is moved by desire to give technical help to the invalid. The invalid, on his part, has consulted the doctor chiefly because he wants to be cured. Yet in spite of the obvious difference between the two motives, the Greeks had the perspicacity to give them the same name: both were generically described as *philia,* or 'friendship'. 'The sick man loves the physician because he is sick,' says Plato in the *Lysis* (217a). 'Where there is *philanthrôpia* (love of man), there is also *philotechnia* (love of the art [of healing])', declares a famous Hellenistic passage in the Hippocratic *Praecepta* (L. IX, 258). Rather than a provision of technical help, rather than diagnosis and therapy, the relation between doctor and patient is – or ought to be – friendship, *philia.* For the ancient Greeks, this – philia – was the basis of the relationship.

But we shall not fully understand the meaning of these two assertions, the Platonic and the Hippocratic, unless we gain a clear and exact notion of what philia meant to the Greeks. Whether they were philosophers or ordinary mortals, what was in their minds when they uttered the word?

All three of the greatest thinkers of the Greek world, Socrates, Plato and Aristotle, found philia a suggestive theme for meditation. Nothing was more important to Socrates than philia. Talking to Lysis and Menexenus one day in the palaestra at Miccus, he told them in a confessional outburst:

I am one who from my childhood upward have set my heart upon a certain thing. All people have their fancies; some desire horses, and others dogs; and some are fond of gold, and others of honour. Now I have no desire of any of these things; but I have a passion for friends; and I would rather have a good friend than the best cock or quail in the world. I would even go further and say the best horse or dog. Yea, by the dog of Egypt, I should greatly prefer a real friend to all the gold of Darius himself: I am such a lover of friends as that. (*Lysis* 211e)

Following his master's example, Plato repeatedly meditated on the subject of philia; and Aristotle could not refrain from saying that friendship was 'one of the most indispensable requirements of life' (*Nicomachean Ethics* VIII, 1155a).

But what exactly did philia mean to Socrates, Plato and Aristotle? There are passages in Plato's writings – the *Symposium* and the *Phaedrus* – in which he establishes a clear distinction between philia and 'love' in the strict sense (*erôs*); but in others he roundly affirms their essential connection. 'For we speak of friendship, first, when there is some similarity or equality of virtue', he says in the *Laws*; 'but it is possible to be a friend to both rich and poor although these are generally opposed to one another; and when these feelings are intense we call them love' (837b). According to this, erotic love is an especially lively form of friendship. We must not forget the bisexuality of *erôs* in ancient Greece, nor the prevalence of male homosexuality in the Athens of Plato's day and throughout his works.

This essential connection between philia and *erôs* enables us to grasp the theory of friendship expounded in the *Lysis,* one of the dialogues of Plato's youth. Philia, the philosopher teaches us, is based on a secret kinship or feeling of familiarity (*to oikeion*) which binds a man to his friends; and this in its turn is based on nature (*physis*). But the need for philia is not completely fulfilled by a single friend, or even by them all combined, for we may always make new friends; and from this we must conclude that a man is our friend in so far as he is an individual part of a primary and fundamental reality – the *prôton philon* (the 'protofriendly' or 'protoamiable' as it were) – something that belongs to the basic roots of human nature and therefore to the nature of the universe (the *archaia physis* or 'primeval nature' of which Plato speaks in the *Symposium* 193c).

It follows that the relation of the soul to the *prôton philon* has two possible interpretations. In a superficial sense, it is an impulse arising from inanimate nature into life, from privation to plenty; and in its deeper interpretation, it is a return of the soul to its 'primeval nature'. Thus it is possible to understand *erôs* as engendering philia, and philia as becoming *erôs*. The original impulse towards perfection and good, in which *erôs* consists, pulses through the very roots of philia. In other words: for Plato, the aim of friendship is *the perfection of human nature – and therefore of the nature of the universe – through its expression in the individualities of friends.*

Aristotle, too, began to make distinctions between *erôs* and philia. *Erôs*, he tells us, has its origin in visual pleasure, and philia in benevolence (*Nic. Eth.* 1167a). Sight is the most valuable of the senses to lovers; to friends, on the other hand, companionship is preferable to all else (1171b). It would seem therefore that sight is the sense appropriate to *theôria* and *erôs*, and hearing to ethics and philia. But after a more careful reading we are obliged to rectify this first impression. *Erôs*, so Aristotle twice tells us, is an extreme or exaggerated form (*hyperbolê*) of philia (1158a, 1172a). *Erôs*, in fact, could be called an especially intense friendship to which a homo- or heterosexual component has been added.

What, then, does philia consist in? Aristotle's reply has definite echoes of Platonism. The idea of 'familiarity' or 'kinship' (*oikeion*) between friends unexpectedly crops up in his compact prose (1155a), and gives us a clear idea of his views on the subject of perfect friendship.

In imperfect friendship – motivated by expediency or pleasure – a man is attracted by what his friend owns or does; but perfect philia is based on what the friend is, on his individual character or *êthos*. However, the three Aristotelian forms of friendship can all be seen to have something in common: the fact that such a relationship always depends on '*what*'. I would not choose my friend for being *who* he is, but for being *what* he is. Aristotle – like Plato, and like all the Greeks – did not understand existence in personal terms, and thus his mind reduced the *who* of an individual to the single *what* of every human being's natural condition (the fact that he could reply 'a man' to the question 'what are you?'), and to those other diverse *whats* (tall, short, fair, dark, intelligent, stupid, etc.) by means of which the *who* was realised. The nature of a thing is *what* makes it be as it is; and this is the reason for Aristotle's very significant declaration that 'a good friend is desirable by his very nature' (1170a).

To sum up: for Aristotle, as for Plato, *friendship consisted in desiring and procuring the friend's good, the friend being understood as human nature realised in an individual*. The aim of friendship should be the perfection of nature. The Platonic notion of philia is latent in the pages of the *Nicomachean Ethics*.

Greek thought could not go beyond this point. Later, the Stoics were to invent the term *philanthrôpia*, and to declare that in principle a man should be a friend to any other man, but the motive for this friendship was still the perfection of human nature as such. To the Greek mentality, both friendship and *philanthrôpia* were always *physiophilia,* or love of universal nature, in its special form of 'human nature'. The Hippocratic Asclepiads, perhaps even Hippocrates himself – who drew up Book I of the *Epidemics,* – said that the natural perfections of each thing conspired together to form the perfection of the universe. It was to the habitual desire to have a share in this conspiracy that the Greeks gave the name of philia or friendship.

Philia, as one of the generic forms of human relationships, was to the Greeks the basis of the doctor and patient relationship, specifically described as 'medical philia' – or 'iatrified', as it were. How did the Hippocratic Asclepiads and the sick men of ancient Greece understand this 'iatrification' of philia?

Friendship : the doctor's view

Let us first take the doctor's point of view. For him, friendship with the patient consisted in a correct combination of *philanthrôpia* (love of man as such) and *philotechnia* (love of the art of healing). A doctor was thus a friend to his patient both as 'technophile', or friend of medicine, and 'anthropophile', or friend of man[1].

We have already arrived at a fairly exact notion of what *philanthrôpia* meant to an ancient Greek, whether doctor or no. Let us now consider what an Asclepiad understood by *philotechnia,* or the love of the skill he employed as a doctor.

What did *technê* mean to the Greeks? None of them gave a clearer definition than Aristotle. Unlike the 'empiric physician' *(empeiros)* who was content to learn how to do a thing by dint of repetition, the 'artist' or 'technician' *(technîtês)* acted in the full knowledge of *what* he was doing and *why;* and his actions might be, according to circumstances, an imitation *(mimêsis)* of what nature did of her own accord, or the creation (*poiêsis*) of something that had never before existed in nature but followed her line of development. According to this, some arts, like painting or music, were purely imitative, while others, like architecture, politics and medicine, were mainly creative or inventive.

Thus understood, *technê iatrikê* is the practice of assisting nature, both imitatively and creatively, in her tendency towards healing; it is enlightened by science (by 'true reason', *alêthês logos,* says Aristotle in the *Nicomachean Ethics*), and therefore founded upon *physiologia,* or the scientific understanding of nature herself. A doctor's function is 'creative' in that he may succeed in curing patients who would never have recovered if left to themselves; it is 'imitative' in that medicine is faithful to nature, and the cures a doctor achieves through his skill in no way differ from those that happen naturally.

Book I of the *Epidemics* tells us that a doctor is 'the servant of his art', and through that service he becomes the servant of nature.

What then did a Greek doctor understand by *philotechnia* or 'the love of the art of healing'? The answer is clear: it meant his love of technical knowledge, because it allowed him to help the patient's own natural tendency to get well, that is to say, to remedy a dangerously altered state of nature. A 'technophile' doctor combined philia, *logos* and *erôs*: philia, because he was the friend of the patient and of the art of healing; *logos* because his skill was founded on a basis of *physiologia,* and because, as Aristotle once said, medicine was the *logos* of health (*Metaph.* XII, 1070a); and lastly *erôs*, because in the very heart of *philotechnia* there pulsed a strong impulse to make nature perfect, and this was what Plato referred to when he said that medicine was 'the knowledge of the loves *and* desires of the body' (*Symposium,* 186e).

A Hippocratic doctor's philia for his patient resulted from a combination of *philanthrôpia,* and *philotechnia,* and was therefore love for the perfection of the human race as individualised in the patient's body: a joyfully reverent love for everything that is beautiful in nature (health, harmony) or conducive to beauty (the natural recuperative powers of the organism), and an aquiescently respectful love for the dark and terrible inevitability with which nature imposes mortal or incurable disease. This is the *anankê physeôs* which the Christians were also to acknowledge later on.

Votive relief of Archinos dedicated to the oracle god Amphiaros at Oropus (Attica). The scenes of the relief show different curative hopes of the devotee who commissioned it. The effect is simultaneous: he is lying down and being licked by a snake, while in the foreground he stands dreaming that the god is operating on him. Fourth century BC, National Museum, Athens.

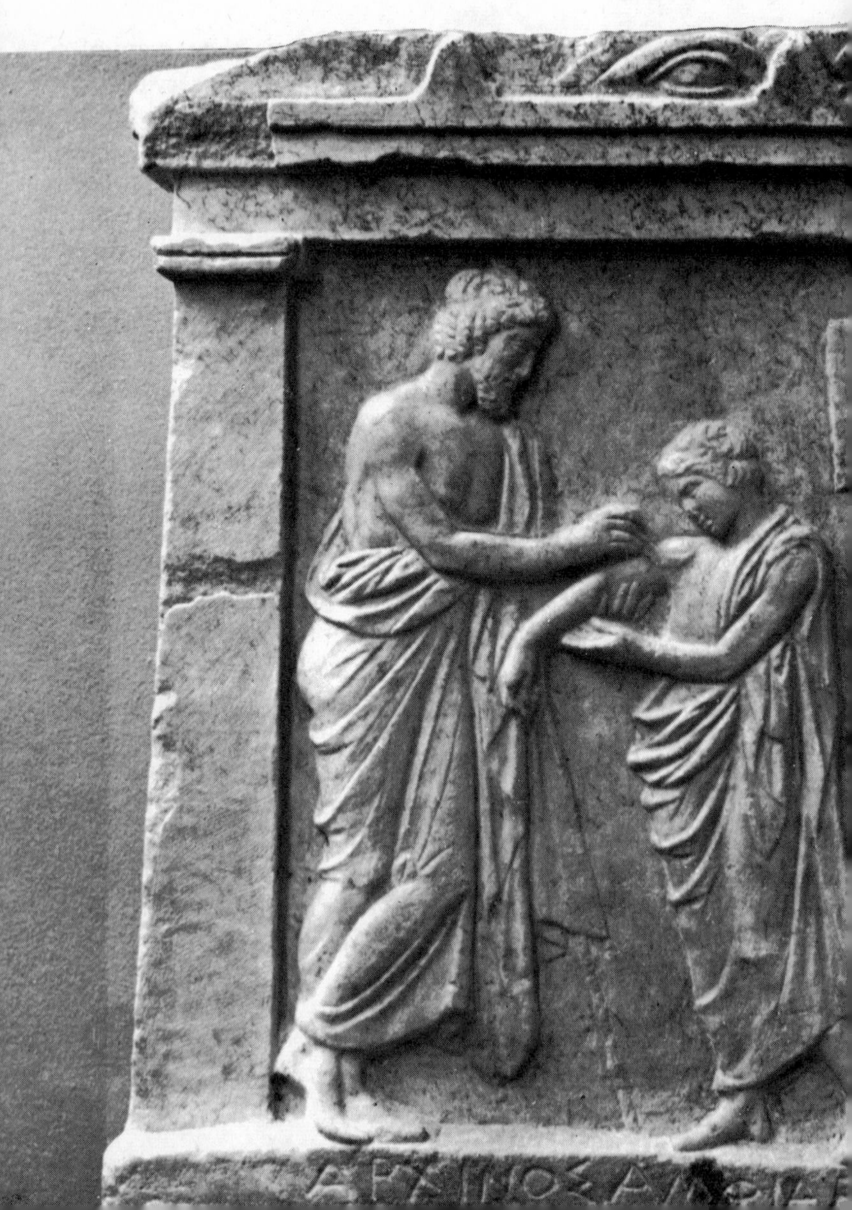

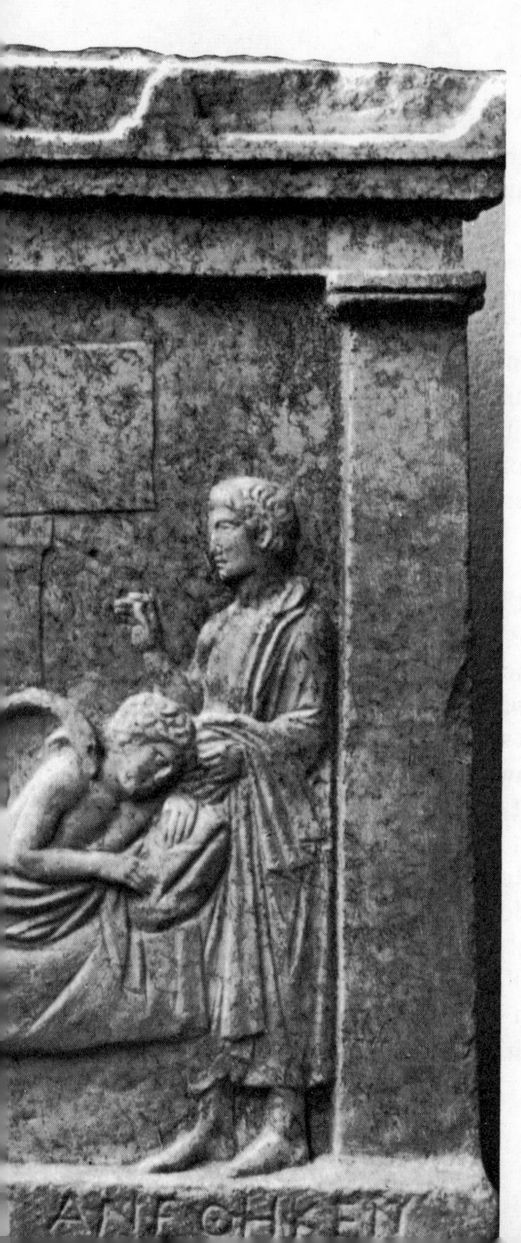

The patient's view

In what sense is the patient, for his part, the doctor's friend? Generically speaking, two separate ingredients are blended in his friendship: first, his confidence in medicine, and therefore in doctors as such; secondly, his confidence in the particular doctor who is looking after him, often followed by gratitude.

A Greek patient's confidence in the art of healing was ultimately based on the religious and sacred prestige surrounding the various arts or *technai* of ancient Greece. The mythopoeic mentality of the Greeks interpreted the origin of the arts as a theft from the gods (the myth of Prometheus), or, in the case of medicine, as the beneficent and divine teaching given to Asclepius, son of Apollo, by the centaur Cheiron. And even when this belief was rationalised, it lost nothing of the social prestige it had acquired from its 'first inventors', as can be seen from the treatise *de prisca medicina*.

But this confidence could not be limitless, for the Hippocratic doctor's *technê* was not a magic power; nor was the *technitês* or 'artist' a sorcerer to whom everything was possible in principle. The power of *technê* had invariable limits, as the Greeks never forgot.

The confidence of the Greeks in the power of medicine was fundamentally limited by their belief – ultimately a religious one – that inexorable forces (*anankai*) existed in nature. Some diseases were mortal or incurable by necessity *(kat' anankên)*, and the doctor's skill was powerless against them. But this was not the only reason limiting a Greek patient's confidence in his physician's abilities. Some dissatisfaction was more than

Votive relief dedicated to Asclepius.
A man and a boy sacrifice a pig to
the enthroned god and to the goddess Hygieia.
300 BC, National Museum, Athens.

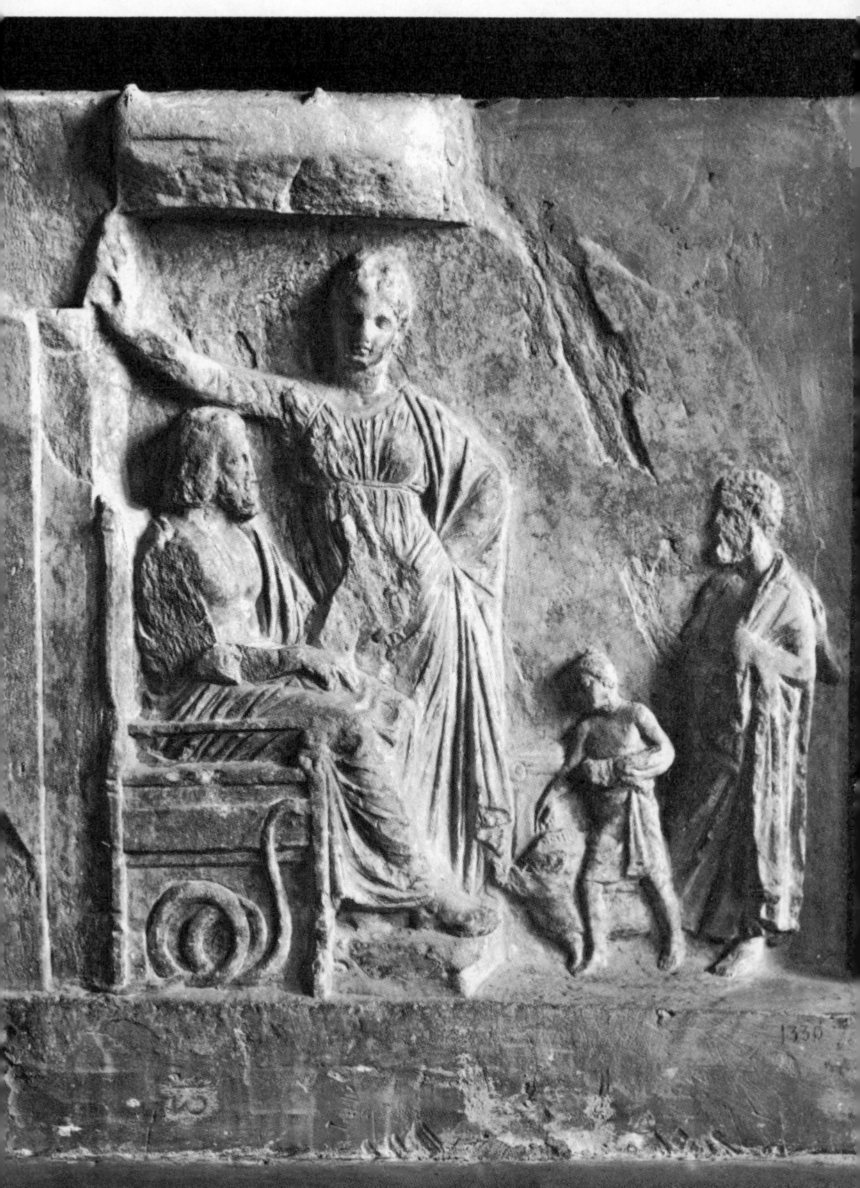

once expressed by the best educated and most critical stratum of Athenian society. In the second *Plutus,* Aristophanes gives us a glimpse of the ironical way in which cultured circles in Athens spoke of the skill of their healers. And in a page of Plato's *Charmides* (156b–157a), Socrates denounces the failure of Hippocratic medicine to understand the part played by the soul in human illness, and declares that Thracian doctors are better than Athenian doctors in this respect. But the Asclepiads cannot have been capable of making use of all the possibilities offered them by their limited *technê iatrikê.*

Technical sufficiency was the chief means by which the Hippocratic Asclepiads gained the confidence and friendship of patients, but it was not the only one. Two of the later writings of the *Corpus Hippocraticum (On the physician* and *On decorum)* describe in minute detail the non-scientific measures to be adopted by a doctor to gain that confidence. His clothes must be decent and clean, and he should be discreetly perfumed, 'for all such things please a sick man'; he must lead an honest and regular life, his manner must be serious and humane; without stooping to be jocular or failing to be just, he must avoid excessive austerity; he must always be in control of himself (L. IX, 204–6). In the second of the writings mentioned above, even more detailed advice is given. According to it, the doctor must be 'serious, artless, sharp in encounters, ready to reply, stubborn in opposition, with those of like mind quick-witted and affable, good-tempered towards all, silent in the face of disturbances, in the face of silence ready to reason and endure, prepared for an opportunity and quick to take it . . setting out in effectual language everything that has been shown forth, graceful in speech . . . strong in the reputation that these qualities bring.' (L. IX, 228). As he enters the invalid's room, the doctor should 'bear in mind his manner of sitting, reserve, arrangement of dress, decisive utterance, brevity of speech, composure, diligence, care, replies to objections, calm self-control, concentration, readiness to do what has to be done' (L. IX, 238–40.). As a complement to the Platonic dictum that the patient is the friend of his doctor because of his illness, the Hippocratic Asclepiads held that in satisfactory cases the invalid is friendly to his doctor for the doctor's own sake.

Medical care in Plato's Athens

The friendship between doctor and patient becomes truly 'technical' when the doctor can realise it in terms of correct diagnosis, prognosis and treatment. This is not the place to analyse the structure of these three essential phases of medical care, but I shall try to show in some detail how they figured in Greek society.

The *Corpus* tells us very little about the social aspects of Greek medicine. The different writings that make it up give us some information about the teaching of medicine, about knowledge of anatomy, physiology and pathology, and about the ethics of Hippocratic medicine, but none about the social aspect of medicine in the *polis*. We have to go to the other sources for this, and particularly to Plato. Inspired by intellectual theories having nothing to do with medical knowledge, and in passages scattered through different dialogues – the *Charmides, Gorgias, Republic, Politicus, Timaeus* and *Laws* – Plato draws a complete and lively picture of medical practice in the cities of Greece. It conformed to the social structure of the classical *polis*, and fell into three main categories, which we shall study in turn: treatment of slaves, treatment of those who were both free and rich, and treatment of the free but poor.

Treatment of slaves A page in the *Laws* gives a succinct description of the medical treatment of slaves in Plato's day:

Besides doctors there are doctors' servants, who are also styled doctors ... And whether they are slaves or freemen makes no difference; they acquire their knowledge of medicine by obeying and observing their masters, empirically and not according to the natural way of learning, as the manner of freemen is, who have learned scientifically themselves the art which they impart scientifically to their pupils ... And did you ever observe that there are two classes of patients in states, slaves and freemen; and the slave-doctors run about and cure the slaves, or wait for them in the dispensaries – practitioners of this sort never talk to their patients individually, or let them talk about their own individual complaints. The slave-doctor prescribes what mere experience suggests, as if he had exact knowledge; and when he has given his orders, like a tyrant, he rushes off with equal assurance to some other servant who is ill, and so he relieves the master of the house of the care of his invalid slaves. (720a–c)

Plato makes it quite clear that the medical treatment of Greek slaves in Athens differed essentially from the treatment received by freemen, and he formulates these differences under three main headings:

1 Slaves were not generally attended by real doctors (Asclepiads trained in the medical schools of Cos, Cnidus, Cyrene or Sicily) but by rough empiricists who had learned the superficial routine of the art of healing from a physician, nearly always as his slave.

2 Verbal communication between healer and patient was reduced to a minimum. The medicine practised on slaves conformed to what was thought about them in classical Greece, and was a sort of 'veterinary service for men'.

3 Individualisation of treatment was therefore also minimal. Patients were submitted indiscriminately to an egalitarian standard; and the healer tried to control the course of nature with his prescriptions, 'like an obstinate and ignorant tyrant, who will not allow anything to be done contrary to his appointment, or any question to be asked' (*Politicus,* 294c). A crude and purely quantitative appraisal – child, adult, large, small – must have been the sole criterion for adapting the treatment to the individual.

It is hardly surprising that the congregations in the temples of Asclepius were largely made up of Athenian slaves, driven thither both by economic causes (poverty) and religious and intellectual motives (religiosity of an uneducated and superstitious sort).

Treatment of the free and rich Doctors behaved very differently to patients who were both free and rich. Yet even these sometimes had recourse to incubation in the temple. If

Asclepius head, fourth century BC, found on Melos. Asclepius was seen by Plato as both politician and physician; it was not worth treating a man who could never again lead an active life, since he was 'useless to himself and to the state'. British Museum, London.

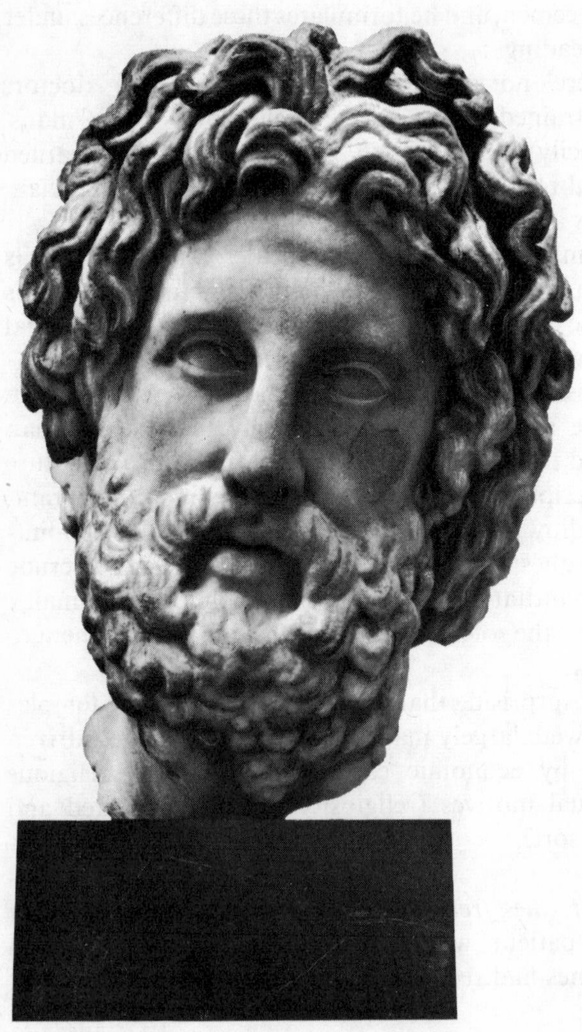

they did not, and sought for genuine medical help, one of the first principles of the treatment they received was its delicate adaptation to individuals, as Plato shows us.

Two theoretical problems concerning medical care aroused Plato's interest: that it should be governed by just laws, and the actual effectiveness of the general rules of the *technai* in each particular case. How could skills be genuinely perfected if every man and every case were different from the next? How could laws which were by definition universal and binding be efficacious when applied to individual cases? The problem of the relation between *nomos* (law) and *physis* (nature), which was the subject of such lively discussion by the sophists, took on new shape with Plato, who considered separately the relation between law and art and the possible perfection of their respective activities.

In the case of the art of healing, Plato believed that perfection could be achieved by rational individualisation of diagnosis and treatment for every patient: that is to say by imitating the behaviour of the free doctors of Athens – the true technicians of medicine – towards their free patients. This could be achieved by three principal means: medical enlightenment of the patient, verbal persuasion and adequate medical consideration of the patient's biography.

One factor which helped to individualise the diagnosis and make the treatment more effective was medical enlightenment of the patient. As Plato says, the doctor 'enters into discourse with the patient and with his friends, and is at once getting information from the sick man, and also instructing him as far as he is able' (*Laws,* 720.). Another page of the same

In the *Iliad*, great respect is accorded to the military surgeons and their skills. Asclepius' two sons Podalirius and Machaon have a command in the Greek army. Machaon is described in one passage as 'godlike'.

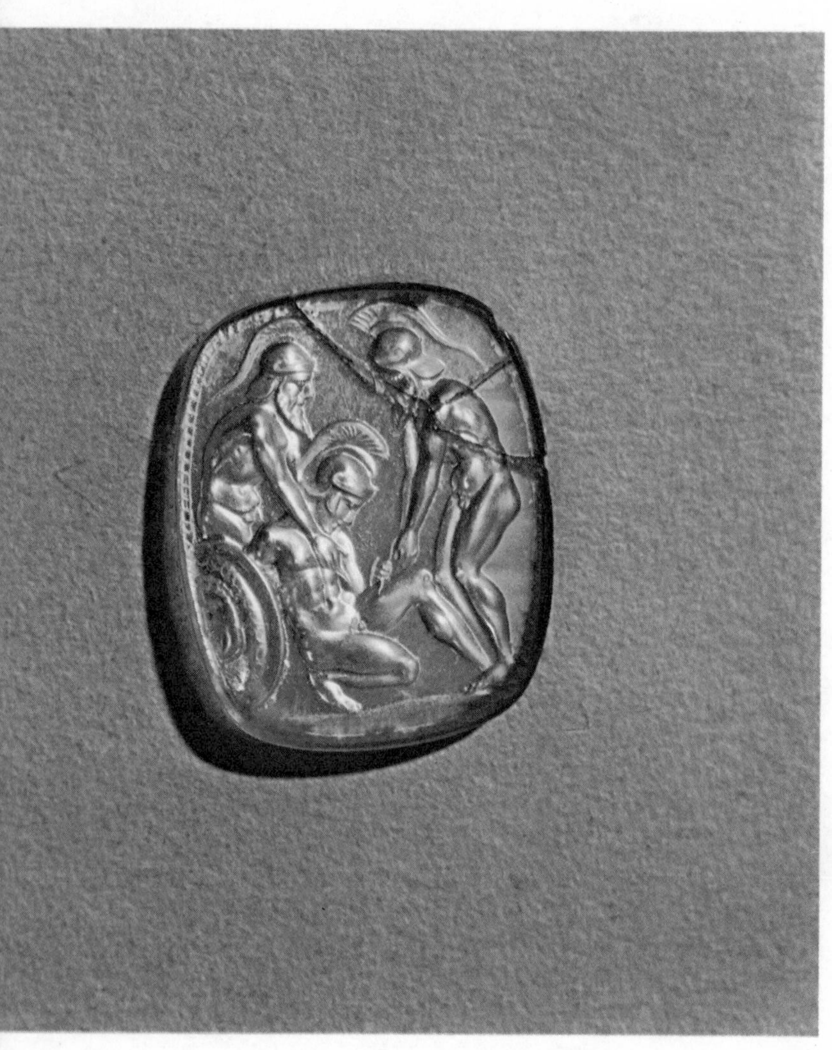

A physician treating a patient.
Graeco-Roman gems of the first century AD,
and (*facing*) second century BC,
British Museum, London.

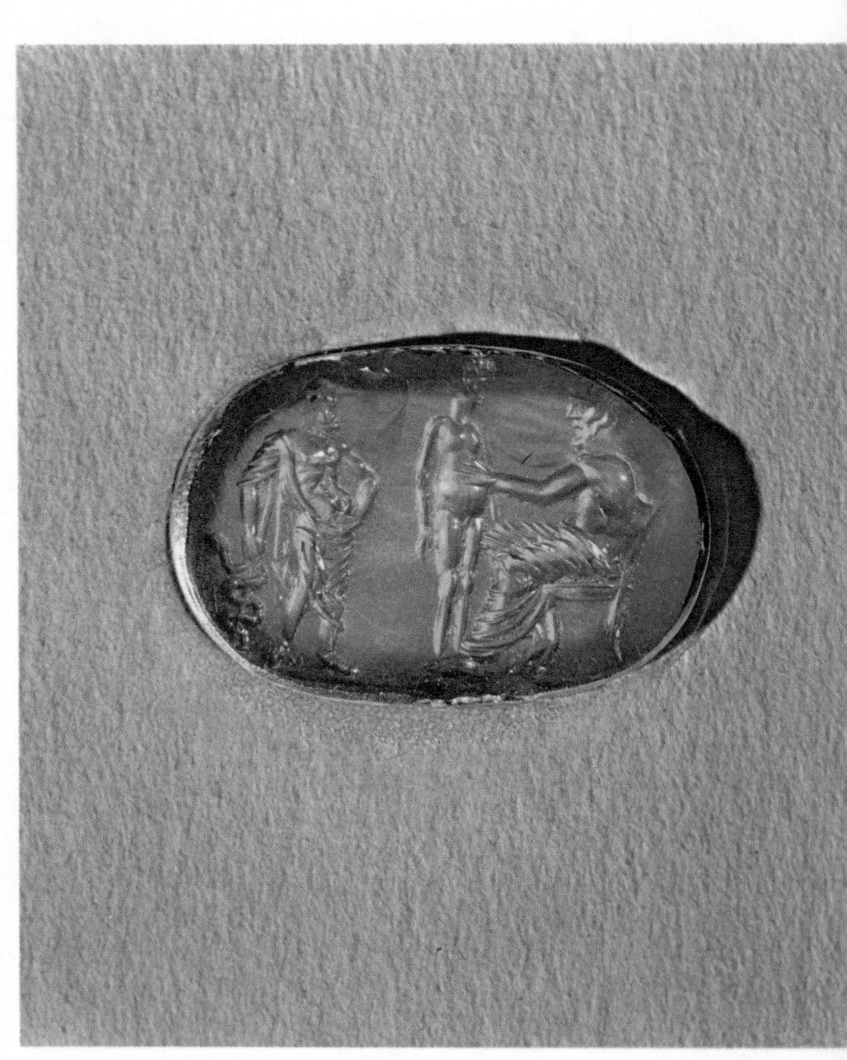

dialogue is even more explicit: 'If one of those empirical physicians, who practise medicine without science, were to come upon the gentleman physician talking to his gentleman patient and using the language almost of philosophy, beginning at the beginning of the disease and discoursing about the whole nature of the body, he would burst into a hearty laugh – he would say what most of those who are called doctors always have at their tongues' end: Foolish fellow, he would say, you are not healing the sick man, but you are educating him; and he does not want to be made a doctor, but to get well' (857c, d).

Plato's lively description is confirmed by two significant texts in the *Corpus Hippocraticum*, one from *On ancient medicine,* and the other in the treatise *On decorum* previously mentioned. 'To learn by themselves how their own sufferings come about and cease,' says the first, 'and the reasons why they get worse or better, is not an easy task for ordinary folk; but when these things have been discovered and are set forth by another, it is simple. For merely an effort of memory is required of each man when he listens to a statement of his experiences. But if the doctor misses being understood by laymen and fails to put his hearers in this condition, he will miss reality.' (L. I, 572–4.) A combination of the doctor's learning and the patient's accurate knowledge of himself helps the diagnosis and guarantees its accuracy. And this is probably the reason why *On decorum* advises the doctor to 'set out in effectual language everything that has been shown forth'. Some medical enlightenment, Werner Jaeger tells us, was part of the education or *paideia* of every civilised citizen.

The best method of gaining the patient's confidence, and individualising the treatment, was *verbal persuasion*. A good doctor, says Plato, will not prescribe for his patient 'until he has first convinced him' (that the treatment will be effective); 'at last, when he has brought the patient more and more under his persuasive influences and set him on the road to health, he attempts to effect a cure' (*Laws* I, 720d). The same lesson had been taught a few years earlier in the *Charmides,* where we read of a pupil of Zamolxis describing the healing effect of 'fair words' to Socrates (157b). Just as the preamble to an equitable law convinces a citizen of the justice of the law itself and individualises its execution (*Laws,* 722c–723a), so 'fair words' persuade the patient that the remedy he is being given is the best available, increases its curative effect, and subtly individualises the treatment.

The Hippocratic Asclepiads did not know how to make the most of Plato's fertile medical intuition. If they had done so, perhaps Western medicine before Freud's day might have followed a different course.[2] But both the unmistakeably descriptive flavour of passages from Plato's *Laws,* and the fragment *On decorum* mentioned above, support the view that verbal persuasion was habitually used on rich free patients in ancient Greece.

The enlightenment and persuasion of the patient were most effective when there was an adequate *case history*. Both Plato and Aristotle declared the necessity of adjusting medical treatment to the patient's biography and the time sequence of his illness, and Hippocratic doctors followed this rule; we need only recall what importance is given in the *Corpus* to the occasion *(kairos)* for medical intervention. But, as Plato says in the *Republic* (III, 405c–d), medical attention that makes much of the slightest pain or smallest peculiarity of the patient's constitution and life history is surely unworthy of a true citizen, as well as harmful to him and to the *polis?* In contrast to what he considers healthy, traditional medicine, man's artificiality and effeminacy have created a 'pedagogic' medicine, whose method is to follow the progress of the invalid's life hour by hour, just as a pedagogue follows the steps of the child in his care. Herodicus of Selymbria, an old teacher in the gymnasium, had probably invented it (*Republic* III, 406a, b).

It is hardly necessary to say that only the rich could afford such a luxury as this meticulous 'pedagogic therapy'. A significant passage in the *Timaeus* (89b, c) tells us that this method of healing was impossible without leisure. In fact, only by giving up all his usual tasks could the patient abandon himself to those who were paying such constant attention to his health; and this was impossible unless the sick man could afford to be idle.

Treatment of the free but poor Between the 'tyrannical' medical care meted out to slaves and the refined cures and diets prescribed for rich freemen, there was the 'resolutive' treatment given to and expected by free but poor citizens when they were ill – for example, the spirited carpenter we read about in the *Republic*:

When a carpenter is ill he asks the physician for a rough and ready cure: an emetic or a purge or cautery or the knife – these are his remedies. And if someone prescribes for him a course of dietetics, and tells him that he must swathe and swaddle his head, and all that sort of thing, he replies at once that he has no time to be ill, and that he sees no good in a life which is spent in nursing his disease to the neglect of his customary employment; and therefore bidding good-bye to this sort of physician, he resumes his ordinary habits, and either gets well and lives and does his business, or if his constitution fails, he dies and has no more troubles. (III, 406d–e)

Such an expeditious form of therapy was obviously socially justified in Plato's eyes: 'Yes,' says Glaucon in reply to this passage, 'and a man in his condition of life ought to use the art of medicine thus far only'. Any Greek of the fifth or sixth century would have said the same thing. The social structure of the *polis*, and the general Greek attitude towards its 'natural' division into social classes make this a topical view, in spite of the dialectic energy with which Athenians discussed the relation between law (*nomos*) and nature (*physis*). However, Plato had more to say. In his view, this way of treating the sick was conducive to the good of the *polis* and therefore desirable.

I do not think it would be a misinterpretation of Plato's views on medical care to reduce them to the following points:

First, in Plato's Athens the treatment of acute illness in the case of freemen was approximately the same for all, and always 'resolutive' in the sense of the word previously used.

Secondly, chronic diseases, whose development depends so much on the patient's way of life, require a more individualised and biographically based form of therapy; this lends itself to use or abuse. A rightful use is made by those physicians who can 'control' the various stages of the malady according to the rules concisely set out in the *Timaeus*. It is abused or converted into 'pedagogic therapy' by such doctors and patients as are caricatured in the *Republic*.

Thirdly, abuse of the 'pedagogic' method is harmful to a patient who aspires to be an efficient man and citizen, and to a *polis* dedicated to the pursuit of perfection.

There is nothing surprising therefore in the behaviour of Asclepius, who showed himself both a good physician and a good politician in inventing the art of healing. 'Asclepius', says Plato, 'may be supposed to have exhibited the power of his art only to persons who, being generally of healthy constitution and habits of life had a definite ailment . . . but bodies which disease had penetrated through and through he would not have attempted to cure by gradual processes of evacuation and infusion; he did not want to lengthen out good-for-nothing lives' (407c, e). In fact, Asclepius devised the resolutive method of healing and taught it to his sons Machaon and Podalirius, who were doctors in the army besieging Troy; and his abstention from practising or teaching the 'pedagogic' method later invented by Herodicus of Selymbria was due not to ignorance, but to the fact that he fully recognised the importance of the *polis* and was concerned for its good.

We do not know what the Hippocratic Asclepiads thought of Plato's medical sociology and political medicine. The writings of the *Corpus* tell us nothing about either. However, it can be said that the medical sociology implicit in them is more 'physical', where Plato's is more 'political'. All the

Greeks believed that the *physis* of an individual human being was related to the *physis* of mother nature, both directly (as in procreation, nutrition, breathing, etc.) and through the society to which he belonged – and therefore the *polis*. Hippocratic physicians could not have been ignorant of this sentiment in their fellow-citizens. But such a view could give varying emphasis to the 'political' ingredient in the relation between individual and cosmic *physis,* and it is clear that for personal and historical reasons Plato gave it the highest possible importance.* A Hippocratic Asclepiad felt friendly to his patient *principally* because he was a man, and therefore a brother sharing the common filial relation of all men towards the *physis*; while Plato's ideal physician felt friendly to his patient *principally* because he was a member of the human community – the *polis* – in whose service man fulfilled his nature most completely and achieved greatest dignity. These two concepts of 'medical philia' are to be found in different guises all through history.

Hippocratic medical ethics

The relationship between doctor and sick man is a part of human behaviour, and as such has an ethical aspect; but this alters according to the religious and moral beliefs of the society in which it occurs. Even if it were possible to construct a 'natural medical ethics', there is an element in the purely medical aspect of the doctor-patient relationship which changes with the passage of time.

* It is understandable that people should speak of Plato's 'totalitarianism'.

The ethics of the Hippocratic Asclepiads was naturally that of Greek doctors, but its 'Hellenism' became modified in the course of history. There is something in common, derived from the fact that they were both Greeks, between an augur of the Homeric period and a sophist of the fifth century; there are also differences between them. Thus, like all *technitai* and *physiologoi* of the fifth and sixth centuries, the Hippocratic Asclepiads were Greek, both in their ideas (theory of man's *physis,* knowledge of pathology and therapy) and professional behaviour (politics and ethics of medical practice).

The ethics of Hippocratic doctors was formally religious. The positivist interpretation of Greek culture has represented Hippocratic medicine as a sort of 'scientific secularisation' of the earlier religious medicine. I cannot share this view. The achievement of the founders of *technê iatrikê* was of course ultimately based on a change in the religious attitude of the Greeks; but this change was not so much a 'secularisation' as a 'reform': alongside the old *religious cult,* whether Olympic, Dionysiac or Orphic, there had appeared in certain circles an *enlightened religion,* whose inner strength came from stressing the divine character of the *physis.* For its adherents, divinity was the *physis,* universal mother nature; Zeus, Poseidon, Demeter and Dionysius were merely popular personifications of this basic and undivided divinity. The fundamental characteristic of Greek culture, naturalism, became a religious and philosophical doctrine. Thales, Anaximenes, Anaximander, Pythagoras, Empedocles and the rest of the pre-Socratic philosophers, were at the same time 'physiologists' and 'theologists' (Jaeger); and the physicians who were

Hippocrates: a doctor should pay attention 'not to plausible theorising, but to experience and reason together'. Statue, fourth century BC, found on Cos and now in the Archaeological Museum, Rhodes.

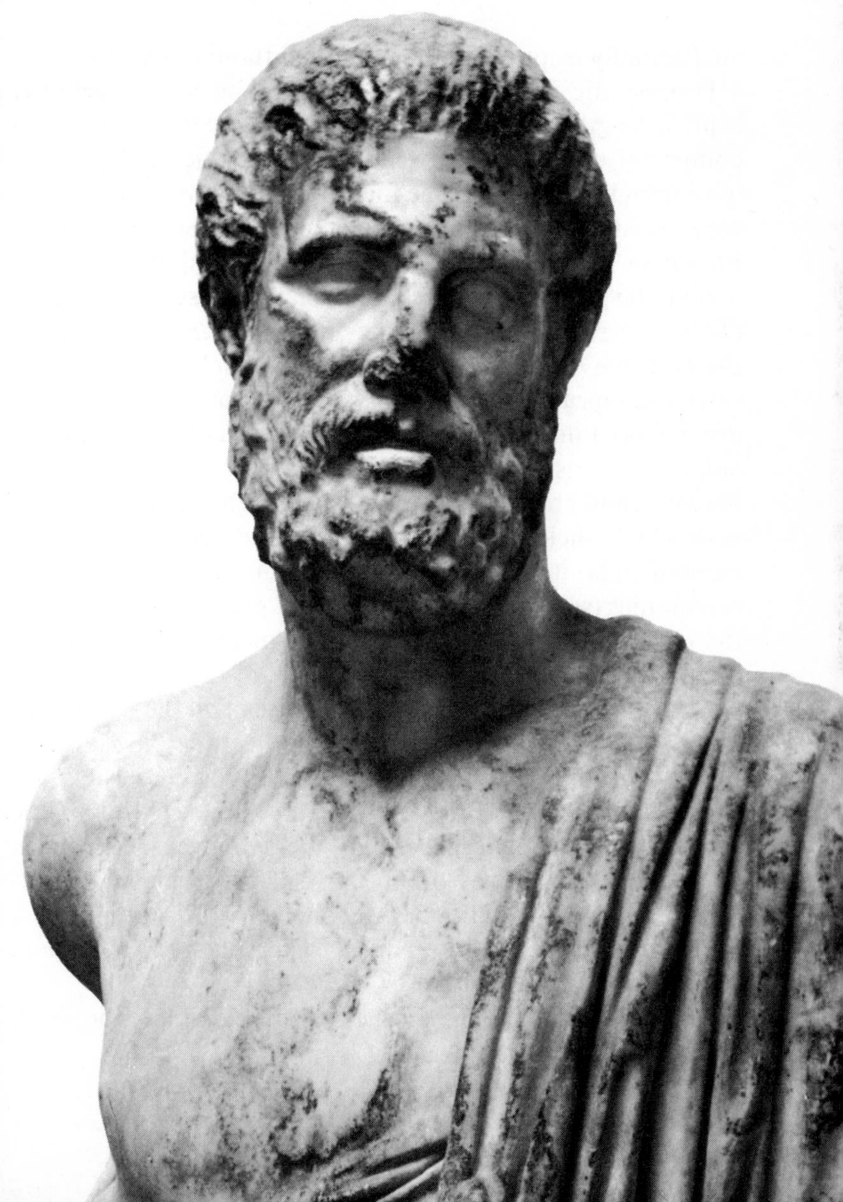

intellectually inspired by them felt and thought likewise.

Hippocratic ethics was thus founded on a very definite, explicit religious feeling, which appears to the historian to be a compromise hovering between the old 'cultic' and the new 'physiological' worship. The former is especially evident in the very words of the Hippocratic oath: 'I swear by Apollo Physician, and Asclepius and Hygieia [health] and Panaceia and all the gods and goddesses'; the latter, in such writings as *On the sacred disease, On airs, waters and places, On diet,* the *Law,* the *Prognostics,* etc. The piety (*eusebeia*) so energetically and repeatedly acclaimed by the author of *On the sacred disease,* is without any doubt a combination of the traditional cult of the gods with the new 'physiological devotion' of pre-Socratic thinkers; it condemns the lustrations and incantations with which ancient superstition tried to defeat epilepsy, and recommends in their stead a combination of religious ceremonies (such as ritual sacrifice and prayers to the gods in the temple) with 'natural' therapeutic methods based on the divinity of the *physis*.

Does this mean that the medical ethics of all the writings of the *Corpus* are similar in structure and content? Some have thought so. In opposition to this view, Ludwig Edelstein has shown that not even the most revered and central of the documents on Hippocratic ethics, the *Oath,* was accepted as untouchable dogma by all the physicians of classical antiquity. 'The Hippocratic *Oath*', concludes this author, 'is a Pythagorean manifesto, and not the expression of an absolute standard of medical conduct'.

Like Edelstein and many others, I think that any thorough

modern study of the *Corpus Hippocraticum* must try to distinguish the school and the epoch to which the writers of each treatise belonged. However, this does not affect the fact that all the authors were alike in being Greeks, technicians and doctors, so that any discriminating analysis must be completed by a comparative and systematic study, designed to show what common Greek factor is shared by all the writings of the *Corpus*, in spite of differences of period and school – Cos or Cnidus, humoralism or pneumatism, the age of Pericles or later Hellenism. Except for slight shades of difference, what I have said so far is valid for all the clinical or doctrinal treatises of the *Corpus*. What, therefore, were the chief ethical precepts of Hippocratic medicine concerning the relationship between doctor and patient? How did the 'medical philia' of the Greek Asclepiads express itself in ethical terms?

In three ways, as it seems to me: by technicalisation of the instinct to help; by an ethical (rather than purely technical) conception of the scope of the art of healing; and by the doctor's attitude towards remuneration for his services. To take these in turn:

1 There is an 'instinct to help' at work in human nature, moving a man to succour the sick, an instinct which is only effective when someone who is perfectly free to reject it – as the priest and the Levite did in the parable of the Good Samaritan – accepts it and fulfils it in his own way. The most central and admirable tenet of Hippocratic medical ethics consists in *accepting, interpreting and technically implementing this instinct to help the sick*. There are some arts, says the

author of the treatise *On breaths* 'which to those that possess them are painful, but to those that use them are helpful', and medicine is one of these. The physician 'sees terrible sights, touches unpleasant things, and the misfortunes of others brings a harvest of sorrows that are peculiarly his; but the sick by means of the art rid themselves of the worst of evils, suffering, pain and death' (L. VI, 90). The famous principle of 'favour without prejudice' (L. II, 634) and the often repeated statement that it is the doctor's duty to devote himself earnestly and conscientiously to the patient's welfare, in the interests not only of the patient's health, but also his 'good appearance' – the physician must act 'on behalf of the good health and the good appearance of the patient who consults him' (L. IX, 258) – are direct expressions of this noble moral attitude.

These methods had their roots in the doctor's *philanthrôpia,* or love of man as such. A Hippocratic Asclepiad who lived up to this moral standard would love his own art through his love of man, and love man – his patient – through his love of his art. As I have shown, this injunction comes from one of the latest of the treatises to be written, when the Stoic philosophers had already spread the idea and word *philanthrôpia* through the Hellenistic world. But the intellectual and ethical estimate of 'man's nature' implicit in even the earliest documents among the *Corpus Hippocraticum* foreshadowed the idea of this philia towards man as such. As a physician and a Greek, Hippocrates was a 'philanthropist' *avant la lettre*.

2 This extremely noble task of accepting, interpreting and implementing the instinct to help the sick had in fact two

A surgeon tending Aeneas,
from a fresco at Pompeii.
National Museum, Naples.

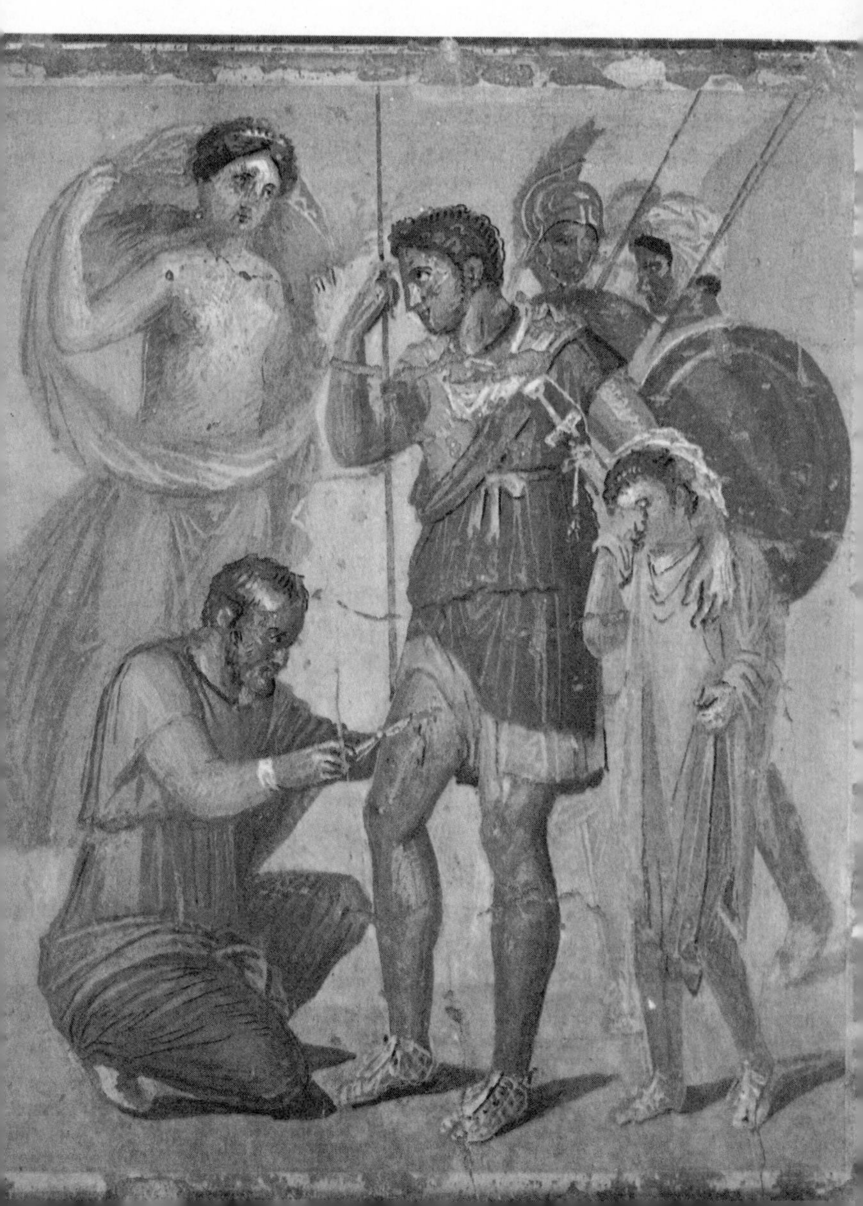

sources: on the one hand it was technical, whence its imperishable influence on all physicians who have inherited the Greek message; on the other hand it was an adaptation of the Greek concept of friendship and technique. So that friendship (philia), whether medical or no, always remained *physiophilia* or love of nature to the Greeks, while technique (*technê*) was the rational skill to do whatever nature allowed. And since *physis* was 'divinity' to a Hippocratic doctor, he was deeply and spontaneously conscious of the religious and ethical imperative to respect the limits of his art, in other words to abstain from trying to cure when 'natural necessity' (*anankê physeôs*) made it impossible.

Nothing reveals this more clearly than the definition of the *technê iatrikê* in the treatise *The Art*: 'In general terms, it is to do away with the sufferings of the sick, to lessen the violence of their diseases, and to refuse to treat those who are overmastered by their diseases, realising that in such cases medicine is powerless' (L. VI, 4–6). The frequency and sternness with which this injunction to abstain from therapy is formulated in the *Corpus Hippocraticum* (*The Law* L. IV, 638–40; *Diseases* I L. VII, 640; *Prorrhetic* II, L. IX, 26), clearly shows that it was not a mere piece of technical advice, but a religious and ethical injunction. Under the influence of his beliefs about nature, man and his own art, the Greek physician understood that it was his duty to abstain from treating the incurably and mortally ill, or rather those patients whom his ability to discriminate technically between 'necessary illness' (*nosos kat' anankên*) and 'accidental illness' (*nosos kata tychên*) led him to believe were incurable or doomed by inexorable decree of divine nature. Even in the third century AD, Origen, in a dispute with Celsus, could still speak of 'persons whom, as leading improper lives, no wise physician [that is to say, one of the Asclepiads of ancient Greece] would wish to heal' (*Contra Celsum,* III, 25).

Finally we have to deal with an ethical attitude that was common to the whole Greek nation. It was what caused Plato to praise 'resolutive medicine', as we have already seen. It was the basis also for the pronouncement of Pausanias in the *Symposium* on granting favours ('There is dishonour in yielding to the evil, or in an evil manner; but there is honour in yielding to the good, or in an honourable manner'), and the later application of the same rule to medicine by Eryximachus ('The bad elements and the elements of disease are not to be indulged, but discouraged'; *Symposium,* 186b, c). Lastly it was the source of Aristotle's advice to abandon a man whose illness was said to be incurable, because he would never again be capable of philia (*Nic. Eth.* 1165b). The radical naturalism of Greek thought, and the resulting concept of *philanthrôpia* as *physiophilia,* had to be expressed thus; to see things in any other light would have been to commit the sin of *hubris,* or lack of humility before the inflexible divinity of the *physis*. To sum up: the Hippocratic physician was the 'friend of his patient' because he was, even more fundamentally, the 'friend of nature'; and he was 'the friend of his art' – the art of healing in his case – insofar as nature permitted him to show his respect and reverence as a 'physiologist'.

3 It is a popular belief that 'charity begins at home' but this

Alexander the Great and his doctor. During an illness, Alexander hears from Parmenion that his physician is going to poison him, but nevertheless drinks from the man's cup and hands him Parmenion's letter. Alexander's recovery vindicates the doctor. This episode, seen here in an eighteenth-century context, points the moral that great souls are above suspecting others.

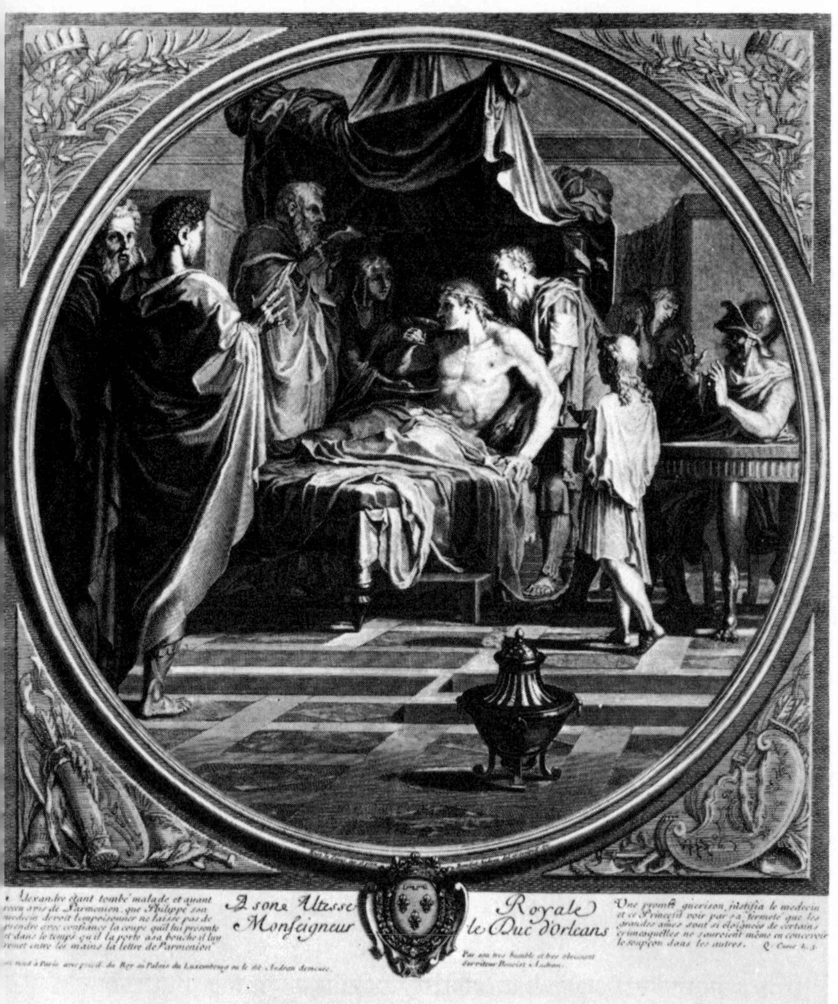

saying can either be given a noble significance (as when a man shows his love of himself by sacrificing himself for others) or an immoral one (when his love of self makes him deny himself to others, or put his own interests first). It would be equally true to say that love of nature – *physiophilia* – properly understood should begin with self-love, and that there can be either a high-minded version of this sentiment (like Aristotle's *philautos* – the man who shows proper self-love by sacrificing himself willingly for his friends), or a less noble or even detestable form (such as is shown by the man who always puts his own fame and profit first in his dealings with others). The last version seems to have been generally adopted by the Greek Asclepiads, to judge from what the *Corpus* tells us about doctors' fees, and also by Greek opinion on the same theme. In Greece, as everywhere else, reality is always notoriously inferior to ideals and to myths.

To judge by the *Corpus Hippocraticum,* the economic relation between a Greek Asclepiad and his patient conformed to the following principles:

First, the doctor must above all be the 'servant of his art' (L. II, 636), and through service to his art he must serve nature. His fees are therefore ethically justified when his professional conduct leads to perfection in the art he practises. 'Overlook the reward, except from the desire that makes a man ready to learn' is one of the dictates of the *Praecepta* (L. IX, 258). A good doctor should always be ready to learn what nature teaches him through his art, and what his art teaches him about nature.

Secondly, a practising doctor should take his patient's economic situation into account, not only because there is one medicine 'for the rich' and another 'for the poor' (*On diet,* III, L. VI, 594–606), but also in order to graduate the fee he asks. 'Consider carefully your patient's superabundance or means', is the explicit advice given in the *Praecepta,* though of course he must not be too exacting, nor 'inhuman' (L. IX, 258).

Thirdly, sometimes the doctor will give his services free, in recognition of a favour received, or to gain a good reputation; and this is most likely to happen when the patient is a foreigner and poor. Because – and here is the passage where the famous sentiment is first uttered – 'where there is love of man, there is also love of the art' (L. IX, 258).

Free treatment of the sick had two main motives for a Hippocratic Asclepiad: one (immediate and interested) was the desire for fame; the other (far-seeing and altruistic) was love of man, and therefore love of nature – in fact 'physiophilic philanthropy'. But this last motive does not seem to have had great social effect, at least in the Athens of Aristophanes. In the second *Plutus,* the great dramatist shows us Chremylus, a poor peasant who follows the instructions of the oracle by trying to cure the god of riches of his affliction of blindness. He looks for a competent doctor, and informs the audience of his failure to find one in these significant words: 'How can I find one? Where there is no reward there is no skill.' The Athenian Asclepiads of the fifth century were a long way from accepting the precept that another Greek of the same profession but inspired by a new sensibility was to give to posterity many years later in the text of the *Praecepta.*

2 The Middle Ages

From ancient Greece until the present day, the ideal relationship between doctor and patient has been based on philia – or, to be more exact, the medical brand of that form of inter-human relationship to which we give that name. Let us once more set aside the numerous cases in which this ideal is fulfilled imperfectly or not at all, and see what happened to medical philia during the Middle Ages.

Christianity and philia

There is one thing that must be said before embarking on our theme. Between Hippocratic Greece and the Middle Ages in Europe an event of enormous importance had occurred – the birth and spread of Christianity – and with it came a radical change in the theory and practice of human relationships and therefore in the theory and practice of philia. In my view, the new attitude appears to have four main aspects:

First, benevolent relationships between man and man are basically of two forms – neighbourliness and friendship. *Neighbourliness,* or the state of being 'close' to another man, involves aiming at his welfare solely because he is a man, and therefore without any need to know him or treat him as an individual. This was how the Samaritan behaved to the wounded man.[3] *Friendship,* on the other hand, involves aiming at the friend's welfare because he is the individual he is. A man ministers to his neighbour because he is a personification of human nature; but a man ministers to his friend because of his individual persona, because he is who he is.

Eighth-century frontispiece of the *Therapeutica* by Alexander of Tralles (the earliest Latin translation of this sixth-century Greek treatise).

Friendship thus calls for acceptance of the individual persona, and neighbourliness completely excludes it. Another person, in fact, *may* be a friend, but he *must* be a neighbour.

Secondly, in benevolence towards a friend we must distinguish between his natural good and the good of his soul, and the latter, according to Christian doctrine, continues beyond death and this world. Natural good (bodily and mental health, beauty, well-being, etc.) effectively contributes to the good of the soul (spiritual perfection, in the Christian sense) but is not necessary to it because it is possible to combine a high degree of spiritual perfection with poor physical health (as did St Teresa of Avila and St Teresa of Lisieux). From this it follows that there is sometimes a conflict between a man's natural good and the good of his soul.

Thirdly, beside the Greek concept of love (love as *erôs*) we now find a new and complementary concept (love as *agapê*). *Erôs* is the universal aspiration of nature towards its own perfection. *Agapê* or *caritas* is the free and active effusion of the soul towards other people and their needs, whether they are true friends or mere neighbours; it becomes formally Christian when the effusion of love takes place within God, and is in some sense 'deified'.

Fourthly, there can be no 'natural limits' to benevolence. Although the possibilities of controlling nature by technical means may be limited, some good always can and should be done to friends or neighbours. To a Greek, to go beyond the possibilities of his art would have been to commit the sin of *hubris*; but for a Christian, to transcend the limits of his art with charity is a moral imperative – a 'commandment' – subject

140

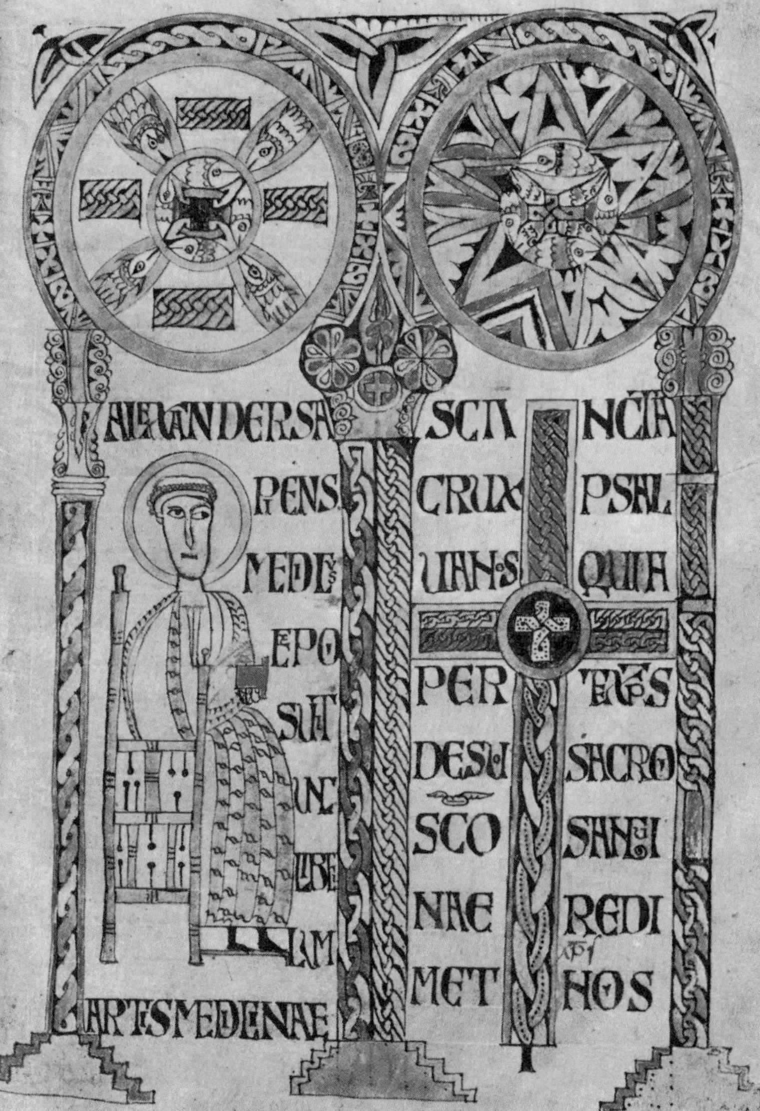

u xx

only to delicacy, that is to say respect for the ultimately mysterious soul of the other person.

These four aspects of the new attitude to human relationships were valid in principle during all stages of the history of Christianity, and necessarily entailed an important change in the concept and practice of 'medical philia'. About the year 350, Basil of Caesarea wrote to his physician Eustathius: 'In your hands the science is especially expert, and you extend the boundaries of your philanthropy, not limiting the favour of your profession to bodies, but taking thought also of the correction of spiritual infirmities' which were considered very dangerous as they might eventually lead the patient to mortal sin. (*Epist.* 189, n.1). The author seems to have read the Hippocratic *Praecepta* and this text shows that the early Christians were convinced they had gone beyond the Greek notion of 'medical philia'. Both love of man (*philanthrôpia*) and love of their art (*philotechnia*) had taken on a new reality: the former for the reasons I have explained, and the latter because the 'art' – medical technique – must involve attention to the patient's spiritual welfare at least in the form of consolation. This led to several innovations in the structure of the doctor–patient relationship:

1 *Egalitarianism in medical treatment.* Medical care was now the same for Greeks and barbarians, freemen and slaves, when they were sick. There is no more eloquent example of this new attitude than the words in which Julian the Apostate praised the Christian manner of helping the sick, and tried to incorporate it in his plan for neo-paganism: 'Behold what has made

the enemies of the gods so strong: their philanthropy to strangers and the poor . . . It is shameful (for us) that the Galileans do not only show mercy to those who share their faith, but also to those who serve the gods.'

2 *Therapeutic and moral value attributed to the endurance of pain.* Describing his life in the hospital city of Caesarea, St Gregory Nazianzen said: 'Illness was patiently borne; misfortune was treated as happiness, and compassion put to the test by the sufferings of others.'

3 *Medical care understood as going beyond the limits of the art itself,* and hence the *inclusion of consolation among a doctor's duties, along with the care of incurables and the dying.* This is dramatically and eloquently brought home to us by the accounts given by Dionysius of Alexandria and Cyprian of Carthage of the great plague that ravaged the Mediterranean basin between the years 251 and 258.

4 *Free help,* given out of charity to poor patients. In his polemic against the pagan Celsus, Origen attacked those doctors 'who only attended the upper classes and despised the common man'. One is reminded of the *Plutus* of Aristophanes: 'where there is no reward there is no skill'.

5 *The inclusion of Christian religious observances* – prayer, extreme unction – in the care of the sick.

These permanent precepts were of course differently applied at different stages of the development of Christianity. There seem to have been four of these: primitive or pre-Constantine Christianity, medieval Christianity, post-medieval or 'modern' Christianity, and the incipient form of social Christian life

A variety of poppy from a sixth-century manuscript of Dioscorides' herbal.

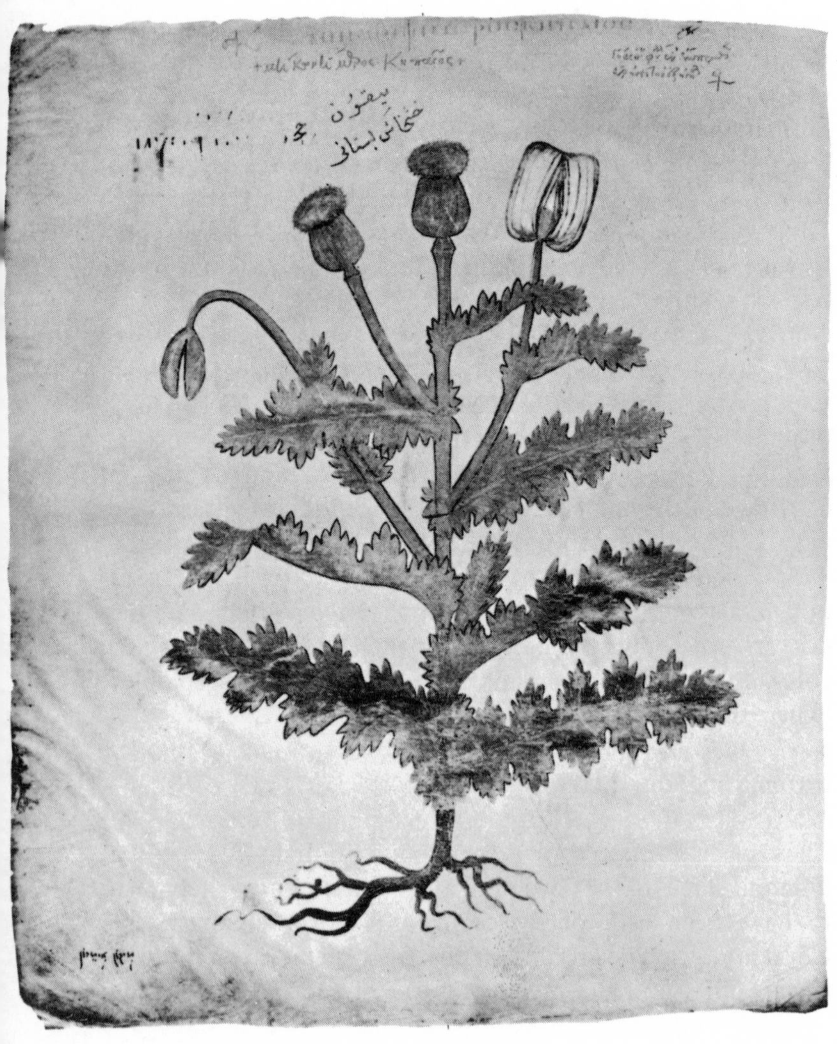

which is now given the name of 'post-conciliar' in reference to the second Vatican Council. I shall go on to consider in some detail the subject of this chapter – the relation between doctor and patient in the Christian medieval world.

Medical care in the Middle Ages

Medieval Christianity in Europe was the historical product of two influences combined: one old – the persistence in a disintegrated form of the Christianity of ancient Rome, and the other new – the conversion to Christianity of the Germanic races that had invaded the Roman Empire from the West, often, as we know, for political motives.

We must therefore try to trace these two very distinct elements in its history. On the one hand we have the structures, institutions, innovations and customs *created* by the medieval Church within itself: theology and liturgy, religious devotion in its 'nobler' forms – Benedictine, Cluniac, Cistercian, Franciscan, Dominican – monasteries, cathedrals and canon law. On the other hand, the structures, institutions, innovations and customs *received* by the Church from the parts of the world that were in process of being converted to Christianity, and *accepted* more or less willingly: Germanic law, the feudal system, trial by ordeal, slavery, and popular superstition. The religious life of the Middle Ages was produced by the fusion or juxtaposition, according to circumstances, of these two elements. None of the manifestations of medieval Christianity – political and economic life, social organisation, science, philosophy and theology, art, popular religion etc. – can be properly understood without discovering to what extent they were the 'creation' of Christianity and to what extent 'accepted' by it.

The care of the sick was no exception. If a clerical or lay doctor of medieval Europe had been questioned about the 'human' basis of his healing activities, there is no doubt that – in spite of professional deficiences on his own part – he would have replied in the beautiful words of the Benedictine rule: 'Care must be taken of the sick, so that they may be served in very deed, as Christ himself'. The first motive for the physician's activity as a healer should therefore be *philanthrôpia,* given a Christian interpretation. But the Middle Ages practised this precept in two very different ways: monastic medicine was purely Christian, while that of the towns was more secular.

There was no shortage of lay doctors during the early Middle Ages. The grandiloquent formula describing the duties of the *Comes archiatrorum* – the head doctor at Theodoric's court and an institution inherited from the administration of the Roman Empire – shows that a relatively autonomous and organised body of doctors existed in Theodoric's Italy. This organisation gradually collapsed and finally disappeared altogether as a result of the wars between the Ostrogoths and the Byzantines, followed by the Lombard invasion. In spite of this, some lay doctors went on practising: the names Guidoaldo (727), Fredo (748), Leo (777) occur in eighth-century documents from Lucca and Pistoia; and a manuscript from Milan tells of lectures being given at Ravenna at the end of the same century in which Hippocrates and

Galen were mentioned. In Spain, the Visigoths soon destroyed the medical organisation left by the Romans; but the *Leges Wisigothorum* proves incontestably that professional lay physicians did exist. In Gaul too, by the end of the sixth century, the brilliant medical schools of Marseilles, Toulouse, Lyons and Arles had been destroyed, and the standard of medical treatment of the sick had deteriorated lamentably. However, we learn from the chronicles of Gregory of Tours and Fredegarius that under the Merovingians archiatry persisted, and various lay doctors were practising, some of them Franks, like Reoval and Marileif, others Byzantines, like Petrus and Paladio. The same trend was apparent also in England and Germany during the early Middle Ages.

During the first half of the seventh century everything changed. Medical treatment now passed swiftly into the hands of the clergy, including lay priests. This had actually begun during the middle decades of the sixth century. In Italy, recently founded Benedictine monasteries – such as Monte Cassino in 529 – started receiving and caring for the sick. 'Learn to know the medical plants . . . Read Dioscorides, read Hippocrates, Galen and Caelius Aurelianus,' was the advice of Cassiodorus (490–583) to the monks of the West. In Spain, Pablo, Bishop of Merida between 530 and 560, did not hesitate to take the knife himself and perform a Caesarean operation. Another bishop of Merida, Masona, founded a hospital in 580 which was certainly staffed by clergy. And although it does not seem probable that St Isidore (died 636) personally practised as a doctor, there is no doubt that Books IV and V of his *Etymology* had a considerable influence on many European priests who had devoted themselves to the work of healing. Soon after this we find both individuals and institutions more and more frequently combining priesthood and medicine, and the priest-doctor became the dominant figure in the art of healing. Many names come to mind: the *Instructio* of St Columban (*c.*550–615), the Monastery of St Gall (from the beginning of the seventh century); the Venerable Bede (674-735); Benedictus Crispus, Archbishop of Milan (*d.* 725); the great chain of European monasteries (Monte Cassino, St Gall, Poitiers, Lisieux, Lyons, Rheims, Fulda, Reichenau, Bobbio, Cremona, Vicenza, Silos in Spain and many more); the School of Chartres.

Three important events contributed to the great transformation in medical practice that began in the twelfth century and developed more definitely during the thirteenth. First there was the reforming influence of the purely medical and preponderantly secular school of Salerno, probably already in existence by the eleventh century; this influence was soon spread abroad by the work of translators at Toledo and other centres where Graeco-Arab science had penetrated. Secondly, the example set by Frederick II's decree of 1231, preceded by the less effective one of Roger of Sicily in 1140, by which it became necessary for a medical practitioner to have an official title. And lastly, the ever-increasing number of medical faculties being founded in the new universities: Montpellier, Bologna, Paris, Oxford and Salamanca. Very gradually, because monastic medicine was deeply rooted in medieval society, the figure of the priest-doctor began to disappear. For obvious reasons of discipline and morality, the Church had

Plan of a monastery, with an *apotecaria* on each floor, from a thirteenth-century English bible. Care of the sick by monks was the nearest many communities of the Middle Ages came to realising the earlier medical ideals of equality, Christian charity, and a treatment that could make up with considerateness for what it might lack in resources.

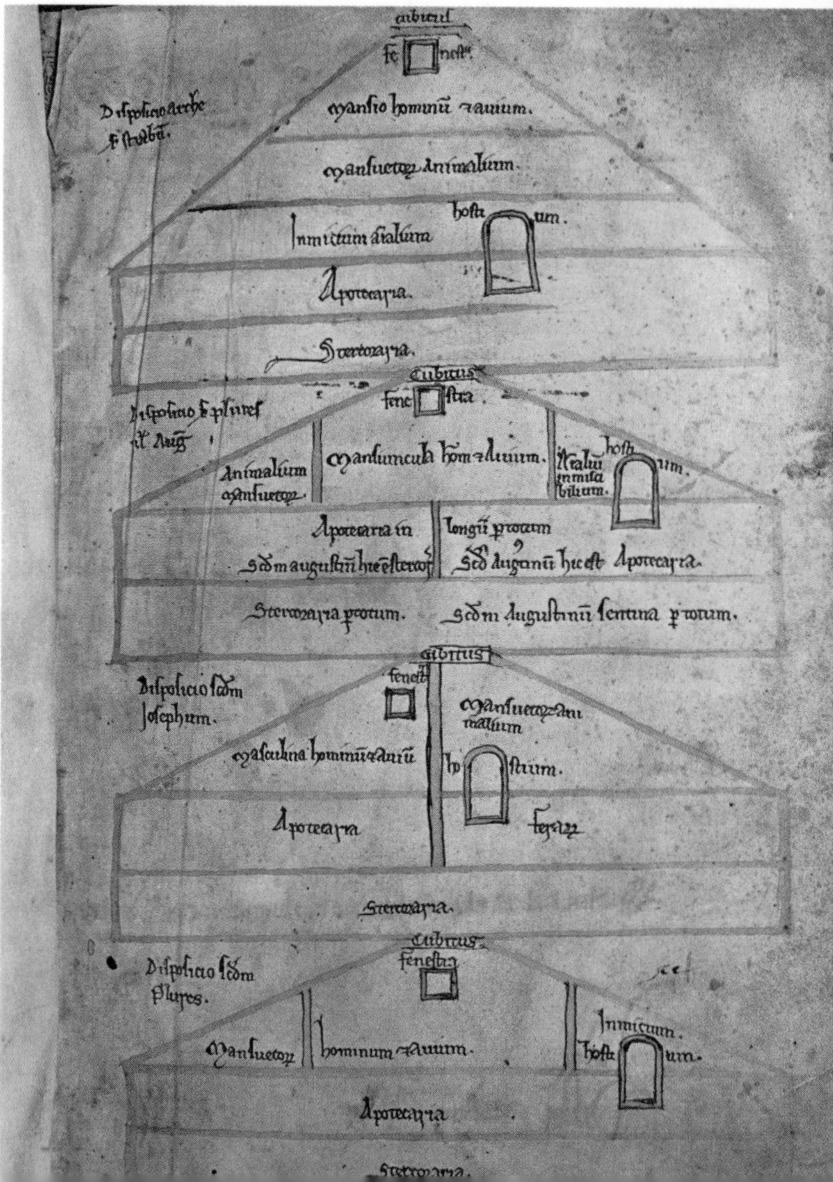

from time to time to forbid priests to practise medicine and the insistent repetition of this ban – at the Councils of Clermont (1130), Rheims (1131), London (1138), the Lateran (1139), Montpellier (1162 and 1195), Tours (1163) and Paris (1212) – shows very clearly the strong hold sacerdotal medicine had obtained.

As before, we will disregard abuses of the system – there was no shortage of them – and try to understand the ideal relation between doctor and patient aimed at in those monasteries where medicine was practised.

We have seen that it was based on a Christian interpretation of *philanthrôpia*. How fully the priest-doctor realised – or failed to realise – the Christian concept of love of man depended on his own personal virtue, and the habits of thought and behaviour imprinted on him by his education and environment. In a good many cases the healer went to the sick man's help out of pure Christian love. Remember the passage from the Rule of St Benedict quoted above. The cellarer, according to another passage in the same Rule, should, apart from his other duties as keeper of the monastery's wine and food, treat the sick man with every care, as if he were his own father. Masona, Bishop of Merida, desired the doctors in his hospital to prepare 'delicate and pure food' for each of their patients, 'until by God's help the sick man is restored to health'; and there is no doubt that many patients in medieval monasteries were cared for in this spirit. Medical treatment was above all an expression of love, and the clergy of the early Middle Ages defended this dedication to medicine in genuinely Christian phrases. Of course this noble attitude often became corrupted, as is proved by the repeated ecclesiastical ban on the clergy practising medicine, from the Council of Clermont onwards.

Among the Greek Asclepiads, *philanthrôpia* had been converted into 'medical philia' by means of *philotechnia, or* love of the art itself. What sort of love of the art of healing can have existed in the monasteries of the early Middle Ages? If the word 'art' is to be understood in its most exact etymological and historical sense – *ars* was the Latin translation of the Greek word *technê* – it must be admitted that love of the art of healing cannot have existed at all during the early Middle Ages, because the treatment of the sick did not amount to 'art', *ars* or *technê*. With the medical knowledge of the Greeks almost forgotten, and the developments based on it by Arab doctors still unknown, the care of the sick in monasteries – and all medieval medicine up to the middle decades of the twelfth century – was 'pre-technical' in character. Rather than an 'art', rather than a strictly 'technical' science, medicine was at that time a charitable or professional 'office'. The monks practised the office of healing rather than the art of healing, for the very potent reason that the notion of *ars* or *technê* was not yet accepted by society. The idea that things necessarily took effect because of their natural 'properties' or 'virtues' – the triumphant product of the Greek view of life, and the basis of all natural science and technology – had been practically forgotten during the first centuries of the Middle Ages. It was in any case not common property; it did not belong to the habitual way of thinking of society. This is proved by two very significant features of social life: trial by ordeal and the conflict between natural and supernatural remedies.

What was the reason for the prevalence of trial by ordeal? It must surely have been some belief that could not be reconciled with the mentality that gave rise to science and technology: some conviction that the regular course of natural phenomena could be interrupted or altered by supernatural means at any moment. If I am not guilty of the crime with which I am charged, and wish to prove my innocence by putting my hand in the fire, the fire will not burn my hand. A sensible and perspicacious reaction against a belief that was widespread in Europe before the thirteenth century is shown in the popular Spanish poem which declares:

Then came the Saracens
And beat us black and blue,
God helps the wicked
When they are more numerous than the good.

Even if God does not help the wicked, things certainly happen in the cosmos and the life of man as it is natural for them to happen, and it is 'natural' that when many fight against a few they 'beat them black and blue' if they want to.

And, besides, how can science and technology exist when it is believed that the practice of religion alone has a supernatural effect which makes natural remedies unnecessary, and that it should therefore be preferred to them? Ever since the dawn of Christianity in the ancient world, and in spite of the anti-Hellenic efforts of Tertullian and Tatian, unsuperstitious Christians knew very well that the natural results of medicine were not and could not be in opposition to the possible supernatural efficacy of religious observances.

No 'technical' outlook could therefore exist in medieval European society until well into the twelfth century, perhaps even until the beginning of the thirteenth. We know that, in the midst of this violent and superstitious world, a tiny thread of light was beginning to transmit from mind to mind what was left of the ancient way of thinking, and that later on this would lead to the 'office of healing' being converted into the 'art of healing'. It is equally certain that those who carried out this extremely important duty were almost exclusively members of the clergy, lay or otherwise – Cassiodorus (490–583), St Isidore (570–636), Benedictus Crispus (*d.* 725), the Venerable Bede (674–735), Alcuin (735–804), Raban Maur (780–856), Walafrid Strabo (*d.* 849), Notker (tenth century), Gerbert de Aurillac (*d.*1003), Heribrand (*d.*1028), the *scriptorium* of the monastery of Ripoll, and the School of Chartres. But, in spite of this, it is impossible to say that medieval medicine had become deliberately and sufficiently 'technicalised' by the dawn of the thirteenth century.

As practised in medieval monasteries, medicine was the Christian office of healing. The doctor-monk used to look after his patients in the monastery infirmary, or – exceptionally – in his own house; in either case the attention he gave them included diagnosis and treatment of a rudimentary sort.

How did this Christian desire to help lead to 'diagnostic judgments'? In the pre-technical period of medieval medicine, when the care of the sick was a charitable or professional 'office', scantily endowed with a few wretched relics of ancient wisdom that had survived the Germanic invasion, diagnosis amounted to little more than the application of a barbarously

Below 'Tironian' shorthand, a ninth-century French manuscript showing medical terms and their corresponding symbols.
Right Page from a French herbarium of the twelfth century. The *hortus medicinalis* was commonly an amalgam of medical lore, passed down by tradition from ancient writers, and remedies believed locally to be efficacious.

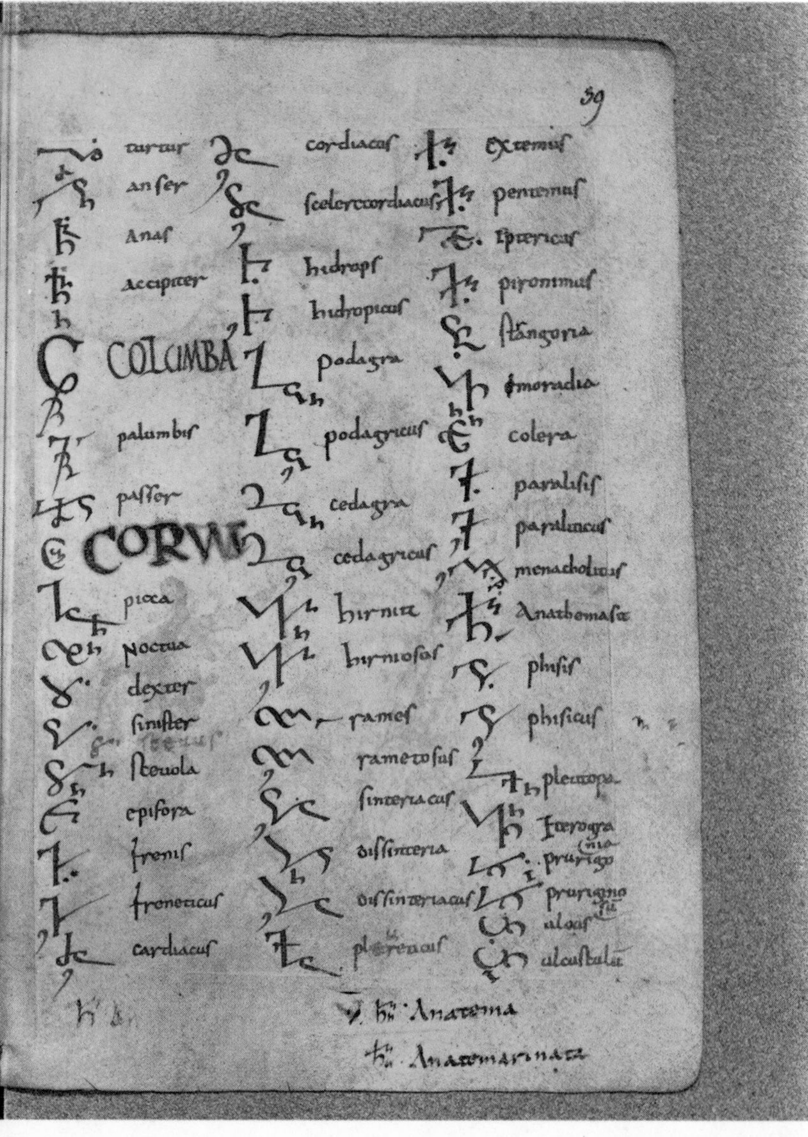

hoc est artemesię nuncupauit.

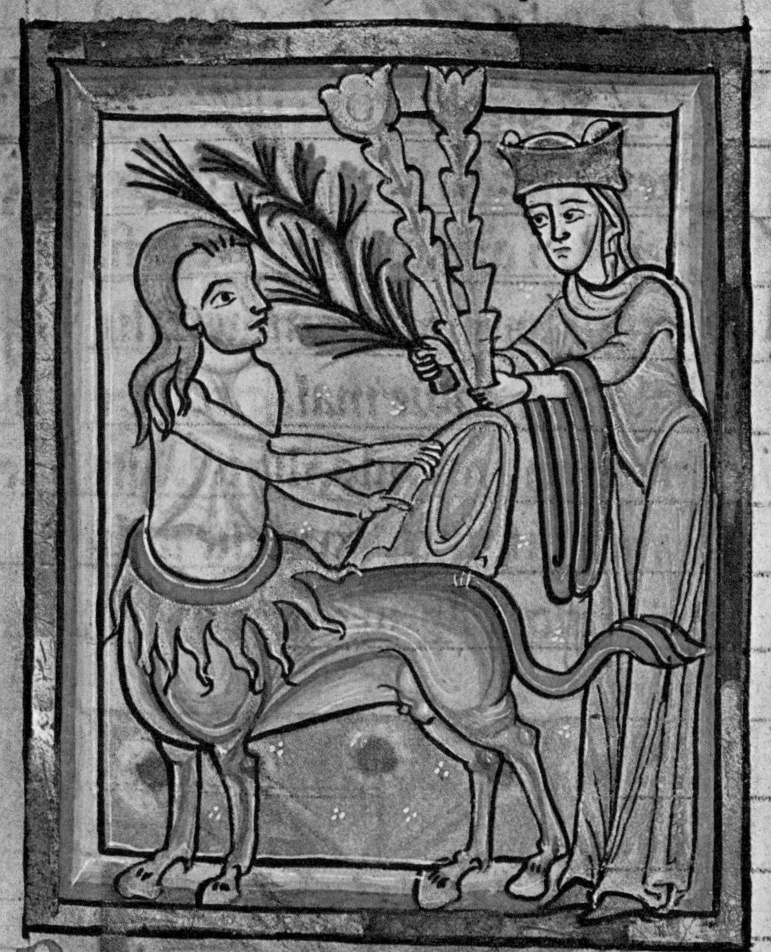

Romani: Rumicem uocant. Prophe-
ematysinos. Egyptii aeuc. Punici. Ro-
micem dicunt. Nascitur locis sabulosis.
⁊ aggeribus ut aquosis. ut circa fossas.
Nomen herbe lapatium.

Latinised name, or attempt at a Latin name, to the dominant symptom in the clinical picture. It is enough to mention St Isidore's *pestilencia, dysenteria* and *phrenesis,* or – centuries later – the small medical knowledge indicated by Heribrand's 'prognostic signs' (*prognostica morborum*) and 'simple knowledge of the illness' (*simplex aegritudinum cognitio*), according to the *Historiae* of Richerus of Rheims; or the more practical and professional note struck by the rudimentary nosographic descriptions of writers on clinical subjects and pathology before the thirteenth century. A doctor used to approach his patient, question him about his malady, feel his pulse, inspect his urine, and name his disease, according to its symptoms.

Then he would go on to prescribe treatment. Care of the sick in the monasteries of the early Middle Ages was derived from three main sources: empirical therapy, Christian charity and superstitious belief in miracles. To some extent supported by what little remained in his library of the therapeutic knowledge of the ancients, the doctor-monk used to prescribe medicinal herbs, usually from the *hortus medicinalis* of his own monastery, as well as dieting, blood-letting and baths. Charity was of course the main motive, and must often have inspired therapy in the form of spiritual advice, or psychotherapy. But the mentality of the period often added superstitious practices, such as the application of relics and various rituals, to the purely sacramental or compassionate exercise of charity.

I do not want to idealise the early Middle Ages, nor to disguise their ignorance and barbarism. But, to judge from such documents as we possess, the treatment of the sick in the monasteries of the time, though so rudimentary from the technical point of view and so close to empirical herbal medicine, was an attempt to realise in medieval terms the therapeutic ideals of primitive Christian communities. Care of the sick in fact fulfilled these three conditions: first, it was directly motivated by charity; in spite of its technical uncouthness it was an expression of true *amicitia christiana* towards the individual patient. Secondly, it was egalitarian: all the patients in the monastery infirmary were treated alike. Thirdly, it was as 'exquisite' in the etymological sense of the word as the economic limitations of the monastery would allow: remember, for instance, Masona's rule for Merida. Intellectually primitive and essentially rough, the monasteries of the early Middle Ages were islands of genuine Christian life in the midst of a society whose Christianity was barbarously and erratically mixed with worldly or family interests – at least in those cases which approximated to the ideal standard. As for the rest, the reasons behind the prohibition of the Council of Clermont may be allowed to speak for them with unquestionable authority: 'They learn medicine for gain ... ; promising health for filthy lucre' (*gratia lucri medicinam addiscunt ... ; pro detestanda pecunia sanitatem pollicentes*). No, all was not Christian charity in the medical treatment provided by the monasteries and capitulary schools of the Middle Ages.

Dagobert, after seeing a vision of St Denis, is crowned king and the saintly relics are taken through the streets. St Denis is France's traditional apostle of the third century. Legends about him are numerous; he was later believed to be Dionysius the Areopagite who joined Paul (*Acts*, XVII). From a French fourteenth-century manuscript.

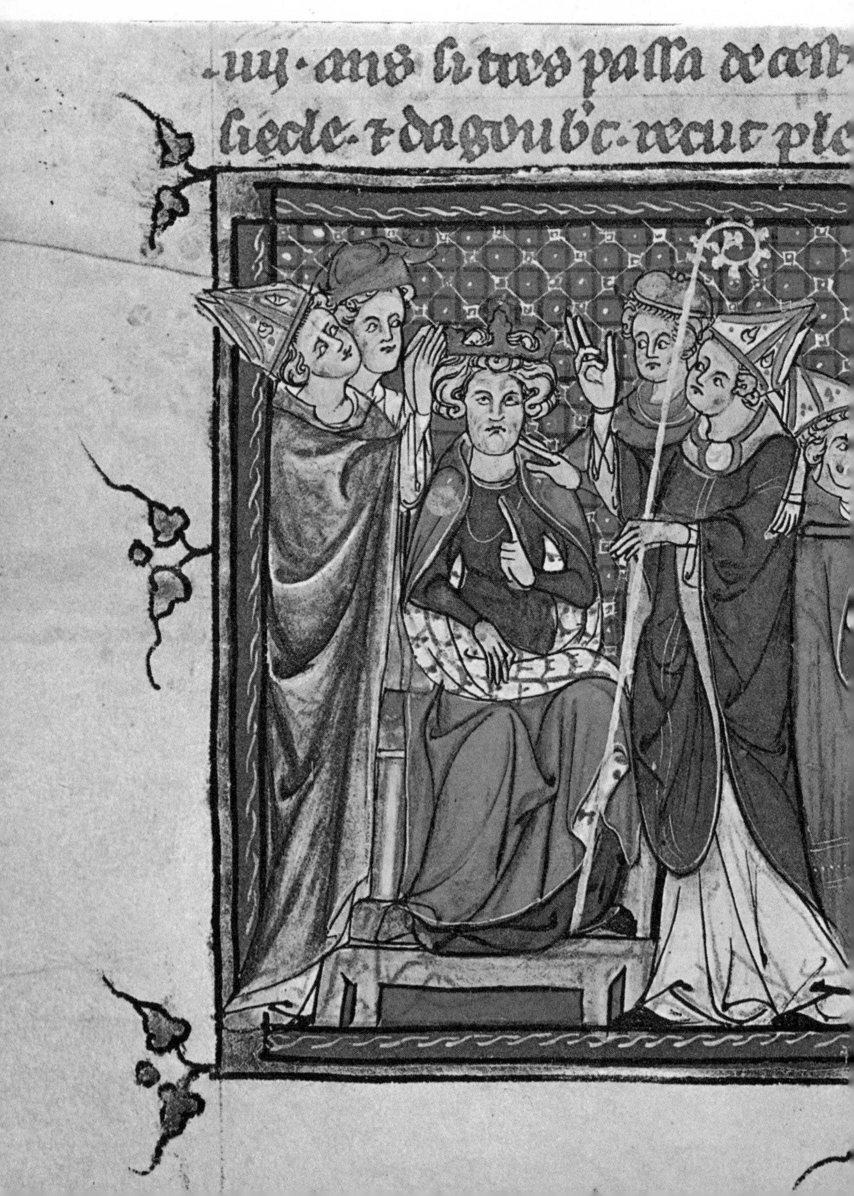

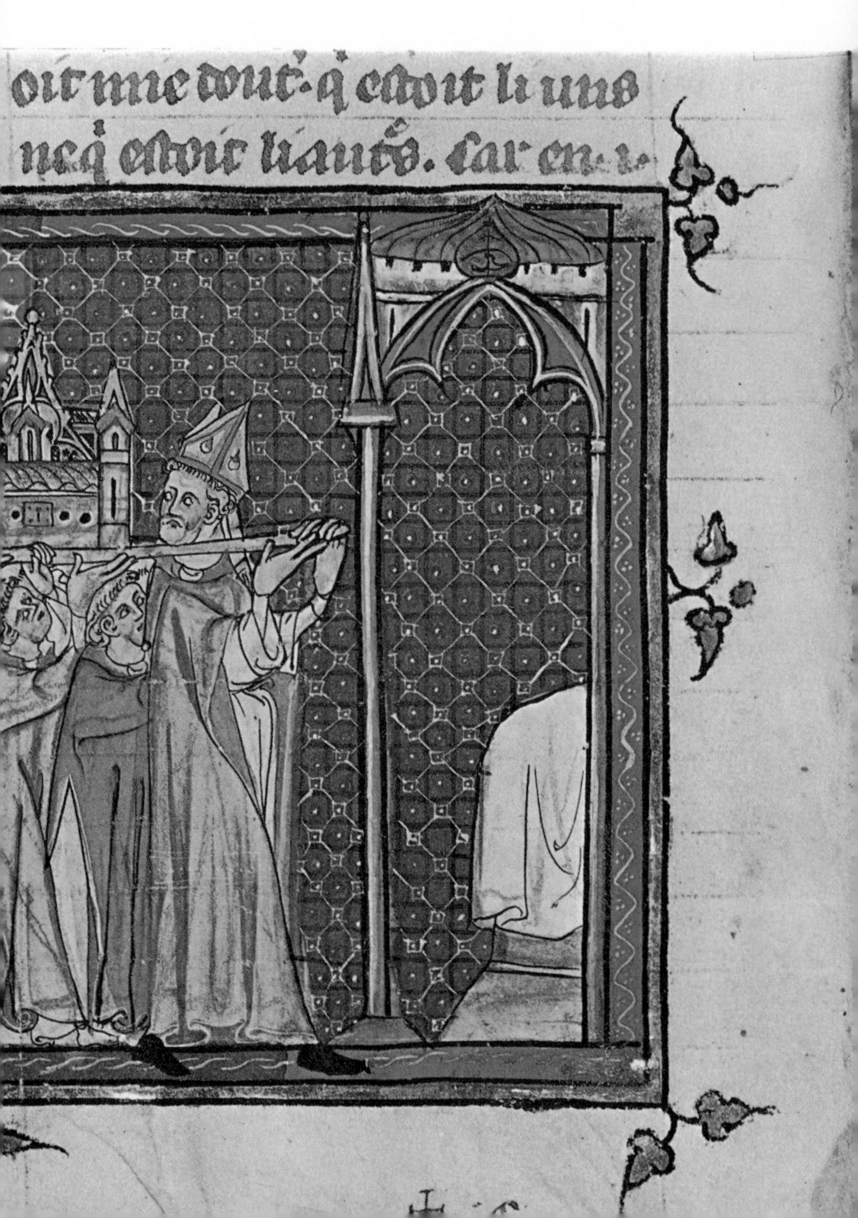
oit une tour· q estoit li uns
ne q estoit li autres· car en

The patient's attitude to his doctor

The secular doctors of medieval Europe – few in number until the coming of age of the school of Salerno, increasing thenceforth, and by the thirteenth century dominating the scene – combined Christianity and professionalism in their practice. What can we discover from documents of the period about their relationship with their patients? How did they realise 'medical philia' in concrete terms?

Let us start by considering the patient's attitude to his doctor. There are two legal texts dating from very different periods: the rights and duties listed in the *Comes Archiatrorum* from Theodoric's Rome (already mentioned), and Frederick II's decree that doctors must have an official title. Both of these show the high esteem in which medicine was held, and so indicate an initial confidence on the part of the medieval patient in the man who attended him. This preliminary attitude often became one of real friendship, as is proved by frequent documentary evidence. Einhard, the biographer of Charlemagne, tells us about Charlemagne's friendly discussions with his doctors as to whether he should eat his meat roast as was his habit and pleasure, or boiled, as they advised. It is no less apparent that a genuine friendship existed between Boniface VIII and his doctor Arnaldus de Vilanova at the end of the thirteenth century. And the abundant literature of the Councils of the latter part of the Middle Ages often testifies to the friendly relation between healer and patient.

But the medieval patient's basic feeling of philia for his

doctor was coloured historically and socially by the peculiarities of the world they both lived in – a world whose outstanding characteristics can be summed up by saying that it was occidental, Christian and medieval.

Ever since the ancient Greeks, irony had been an element in western life. The attitude of the medieval patient to his doctors cannot have been an exception to this rule – nor could that of a healthy man who might become sick – as is very clearly demonstrated in the *Medieval Satires of the Physician,* in which the old Aristophanic tradition unconsciously persists. In the middle of the thirteenth century, John of Salisbury's *Metalogicus* launched a humorous and sarcastic attack on the disputes among the Galenists, with their presumptuously inflated technical terms and their greed for money: 'They make a great display of Hippocrates and Galen, utter unknown words, apply their Aphorisms to everything, and stuff men's minds with unheard-of names, leaving them full of meaningless sound'. Two centuries later Petrarch was to follow him into the breach: in his *Invectivae* he applied the incisively modern phrase *latina mors cum graeco velamine* to the frequent latinisations of Greek medical terms of the period.

But satire was not the only influence conditioning the relation of patient to doctor in medieval times; it had also received the imprint of the feudal society into which it was born, and the 'ordalian' mentality (or mentality of the ordeal) prevailing in it. Above all in the early Middle Ages, although he was a freeman, a doctor often found himself harshly subjected to his master's authority and caprices. No more

A doctor advises a king. Medieval society, by the conflict in its views of his civil and religious duties, could put the doctor in an awkward position on such matters as a patient's confession of sins or the size of his fee. Dante explained the monarchy as a part of the natural order directly linked with the Divine purpose, thus lessening the church's

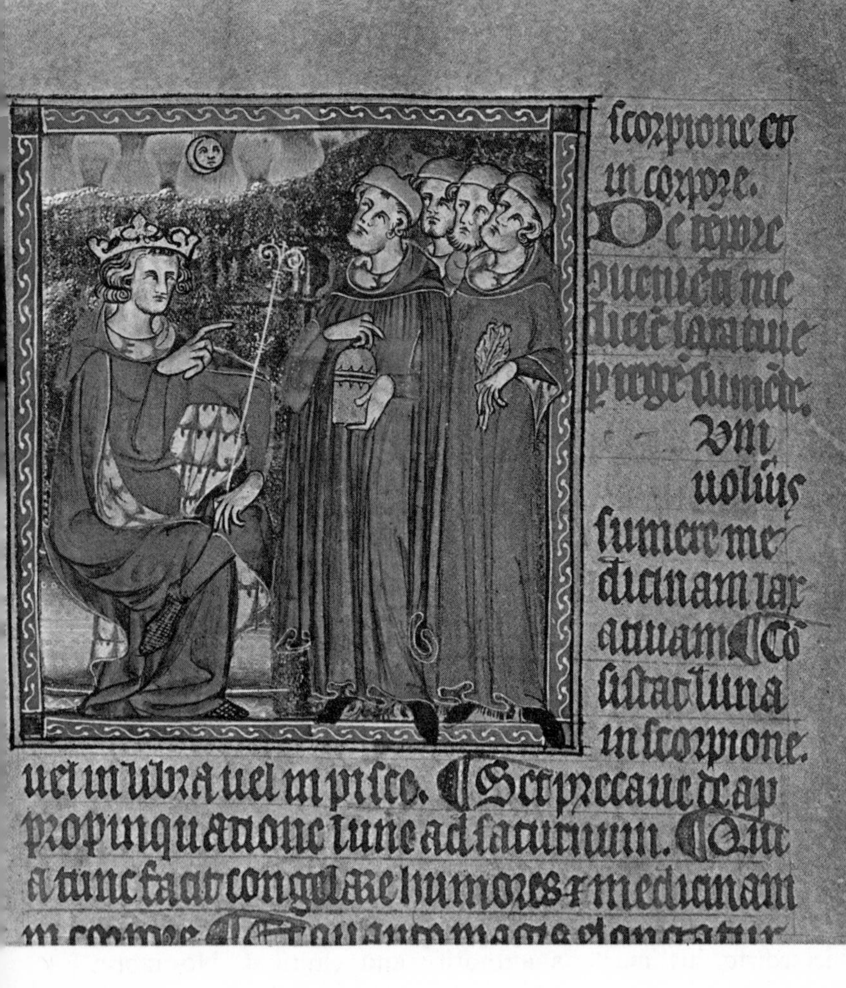

influence. This may have made easier a royal physician's task – but kings and princes were not the only ill people. From the fourteenth-century *De Secretis Secretorum Aristoteles.*

barbarous and eloquent example of this could be found than the behaviour of Austrechild, wife of King Guntram, to her doctors Nicholas and Donato. Austrechild fell ill in the year 580, and aware that she was dying asked her husband to give orders for the two doctors who had attended her to be beheaded, since the remedies they had prescribed had been useless. The chronicle tells us that the dying woman's wish was faithfully carried out, so that the lady should not enter the kingdom of death alone (Gregory of Tours, *Hist. Franc.,* V, 36). Sweet and gentle Austrechild! The behaviour of King Chilperic seems almost merciful in comparison: for similar reasons he had the archiater Marileif thrashed, dispossessed of all his goods and handed over to the Church as a slave. It is not difficult to detect the mentality I have previously described as 'ordalian' in such impetuous behaviour – 'if your neck cannot resist the axe, it must be because you are guilty'.

The gradual process of legal rationalisation of human relations led to the patient's confidence – or lack of it – in his doctor developing a contractual slant. However friendly it may be, the medical relation is a contract and was often interpreted as one by medieval society. The *Leges Wisigothorum,* for example, goes into minute details concerning the possible sanctions to be imposed on doctors. Before undertaking the treatment, the physician had to agree on his fees and pay a deposit. If the invalid died, the doctor had no right to any fee whatever, but could take back his deposit. Technical mistakes were punished in various ways: for a badly performed blood-letting he was fined a hundred and fifty *sols;* if a slave died, he must provide another; if a freeman died, he must accept the arbitration of the family; for bleeding a free woman when no slaves or serfs were present, he was fined ten *sols,* because in such cases 'it is not difficult for the woman to get a bad name' (*difficillimum non est, ut interdum ludibrium adhaerescat*). Evidently tongues wagged and women's honour was frail among the Visigoths! These regulations were collected together in codes and compilations. It was obviously no laughing matter to practise medicine in the Middle Ages.

Finally I must mention the *battle between superstition and medical practice* – that is to say the supposed opposition between natural and religious remedies, to the detriment of the former. In defence of the miraculous cures of St Martin, Gregory of Tours wrote in the second half of the sixth century: 'What do doctors achieve with their instruments? They are more liable to cause pain than relieve it. When they open wide the patient's eye and cut it with their sharp lancets, they are more likely to make the torments of death appear to that same eye, than to help it to see . . . Whereas our beloved Saint possesses only one steel instrument – his will – and only one unguent – his healing virtue.' We find the same significance in the story of the meeting between Donnolo (the Jewish doctor Shabbethai ben Abrahim) and the man who was later to become St Nilus. Donnolo (913–65), who was practising his profession with great success in several parts of southern Italy, had been a great friend of the saint in his youth. Here is what the *Acta sanctorum* has to say about their subsequent meeting:

When the holy man entered the city, he was approached by a Jew called Donnolo, whom he had known since he was young, a very studious man and having uncommon skill in the art of healing. This man began to speak to the Saint: 'I have heard tell of the austere life you lead and of your great abstinence, and knowing as I do your bodily constitution, I should not be surprised if you became an epileptic. So, if you think fit, I will give you a remedy suitable to your temperament which will prevent your falling ill for the rest of your life.' To which the Saint replied: 'One of you Jews said to us: It is better to put your trust in God than in man. Therefore those of us who put our trust in God, our doctor and in our Lord Jesus Christ, have no need of the remedies you prepare just in order to boast afterwards that you have given them to Nilus.' Hearing these things, the physician made no reply.

The attitude of mind of the author of this story is evident. And in the middle of the twelfth century, St Bernard himself was so deeply moved by the desire to glorify God through illness that he became resolutely hostile to doctor's preparations and believed that a higher degree of perfection would be achieved by letting God work through nature.

The taste for satire, the feudal mentality that thought in terms of ordeal, the interpretation of the relationship as a contract, and the popular tendency to combat natural remedies, to their detriment, with supernatural ones – all these factors conditioned the patient's philia for his doctor throughout the Middle Ages. Yet, as we have seen, this friendship continued to exist in spite of everything.

Galen takes a woman's pulse and performs a uroscopy. From a fifteenth-century Flanders manuscript.

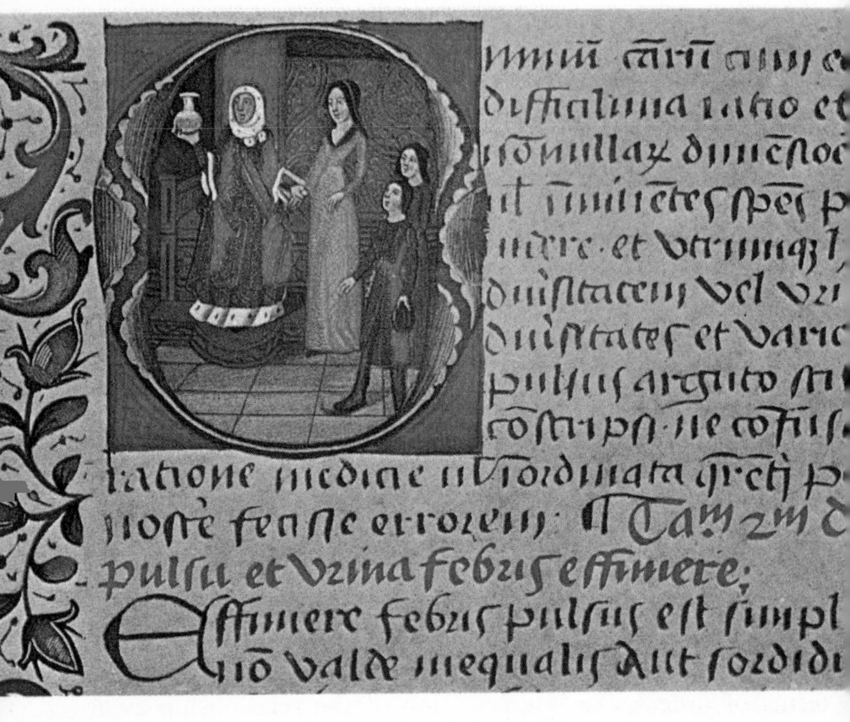

The doctor's attitude to his patient

Let us now look at the reciprocal impulse in medieval medicine – the doctor's philia for his patient.

In the pre-technical period – that is to say before European doctors had absorbed the Greek notions of *natura* (*physis*) and *ars* (*technê*) during the twelfth and thirteenth centuries – the healer was a friend to the patient insofar as he was a friend to his profession, and his desire to help the sick was therefore diluted by other much less noble motives. This is shown by the changing content of the writings of medieval physicians on the politics of their professional practice.

The first of these – the fragment *How you should visit the Sick* of a short *Summa medicinalis* dating from the end of the ninth century – gives practical rules for the proper conduct of a professional visit. The physician should go to see the patient more than once, question him about his malady and the opinions other doctors had given of it, feel his pulse, examine his urine, ask about his bowel movements and sleep. But he also had to observe rules that had nothing to do with the art of healing; imagination and humour were also necessary. An anecdote about Notker, a monk of St Gall in the tenth century, gives an ingenious reply to the satirical view of doctors previously mentioned. Notker, who was known to his brother monks as 'Peppercorn', (*Piperis granum*), had a great reputation as a doctor, and particularly for his skill in uroscopy. For a joke, Duke Henry of Bavaria sent him the urine of a pregnant woman instead of his own; and the cunning Notker, who understood the Duke's style of humour no less well than he did the urine of pregnant women, sent back the following verdict: 'God is about to produce an unheard-of miracle. Within thirty days, our Duke will be suckling a son born of his own belly.' A medical practitioner cannot live by technique alone.

The author of the treatise *De instructione medici,* Archimateus of Salerno (twelfth century), combined rudimentary skill in diagnosis with artfulness, in an accomplished and delightful way.[4] The rules were well known to him: questions, taking the pulse, examining the urine, etc. But Archimateus was clever enough to know that this was not enough to gain the patient's good opinion and conquer his doubts. The important thing was to see that his patient confessed, or promised to confess, right at the start; not merely for the good of his soul, but to avoid his assuming that his illness had taken a turn for the worse as a result of an error on his doctor's part, should he be advised to confess later on. But we will let Archimateus speak for himself: 'Before going to the sick man's house, ask whether he has confessed to the priest, and if he has not done so let him do so or promise to do so; for if this is spoken of after seeing the sick man and considering his symptoms, it will be thought that the time has come to despair of a cure, since you despair of it yourself.' However, the astute doctor from Salerno knew more than this; he knew that it is sometimes a good thing to apply treatment in appearance only: 'There are some sick men,' he says, 'who are intoxicated by the poison of avarice; when they see that nature is triumphing over their disease without the doctor's help, they deprive him of all merit, saying: What did the doctor do? With the aid of his syrups, unguents and fomentations we only appear to have achieved the health given by nature ... saying afterwards, when a fresh onset has aggravated the disease, that it was not the result of the medicine, so that what nature had performed herself was attributed to the doctor.' All this, in a lesson *De instructione medici,* beginning with the words: 'Thus, oh doctor, when you are called by a sick man, ask for help in the name of God' (*Cum igitur, o medice, ad aegrotum vocaberis adiutorium sit in nomine Domini!*).

As medieval society gradually matured intellectually and politically under the rapidly growing influence of Graeco-Arab science and medicine, it began to develop a climate of opinion which helped transform the 'office of healing' into the 'art of healing', and so into scientific medicine. During the twelfth century the intellectual standard of writers increased, and scientific institutions proliferated and became more influential. It is enough to mention the names of St Anselm, Lanfranc and Abelard, and the medical writings of St Hildegard and the masters of Salerno. The medieval intellect was reaching its highest point of development, formed by the new universities and personified in St Albertus Magnus, St Thomas Aquinas, St Bonaventure, Duns Scotus, Roger Bacon and Vincent of Beauvais. The birth of true natural science became possible; and western medicine, with practically all ancient and Arab learning at its disposal, became in the full sense of the word *ars medica,* 'the art of healing', as Taddeo Alderotti, Arnaldus de Vilanova, the great surgeons of the fourteenth century, Pietro d'Abano, Gentile da Foligno, Bartolommeo Montagnana, Mondino de Luzzi and many others were to prove in their practice and writings.

Two events in ordinary non-professional life, among others of similar significance, furnish eloquent proof of the changes that had taken place in attitudes. The first was the formal condemnation of the system of ordeal in 1216 by the Lateran Council. A few years later, Frederick II, who was not a philosopher but a discriminating and enlightened man of the

A thirteenth-century satirical drawing of an ape taking the pulse and carrying out the uroscopy for his human patient. From the Metz Pontifical, France.

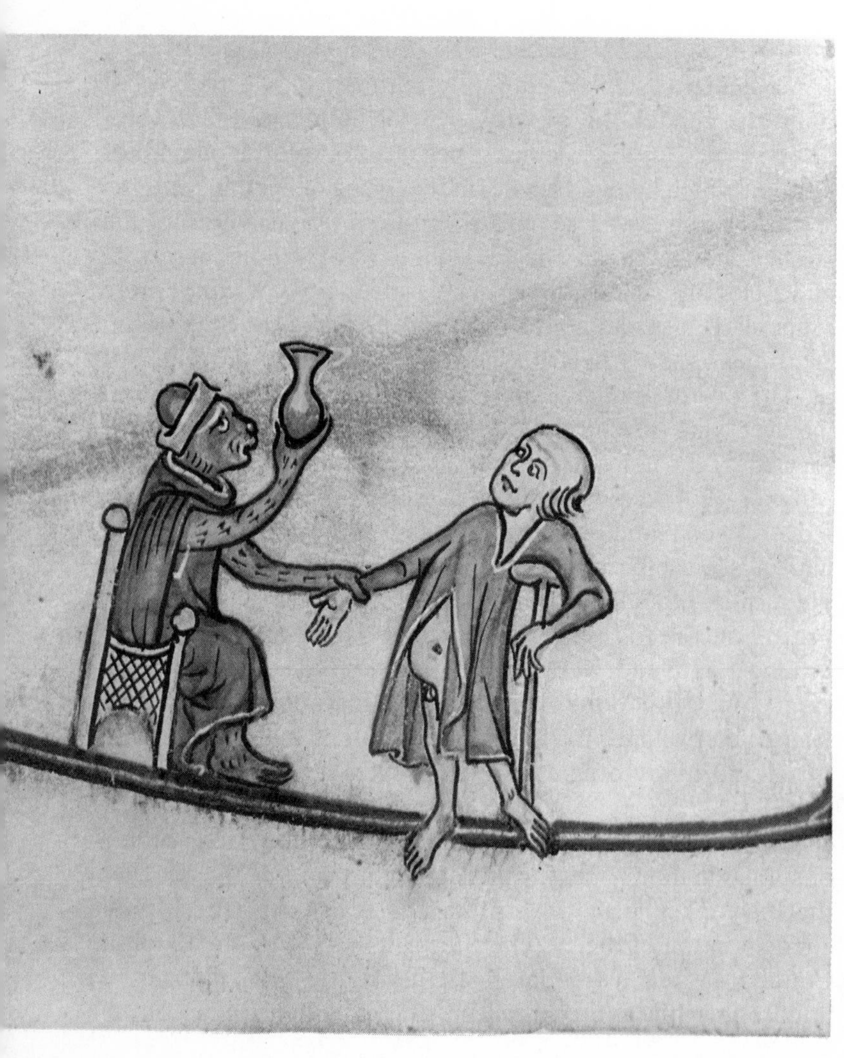

A doctor taking a pulse.
From a fourteenth-century
English manuscript.

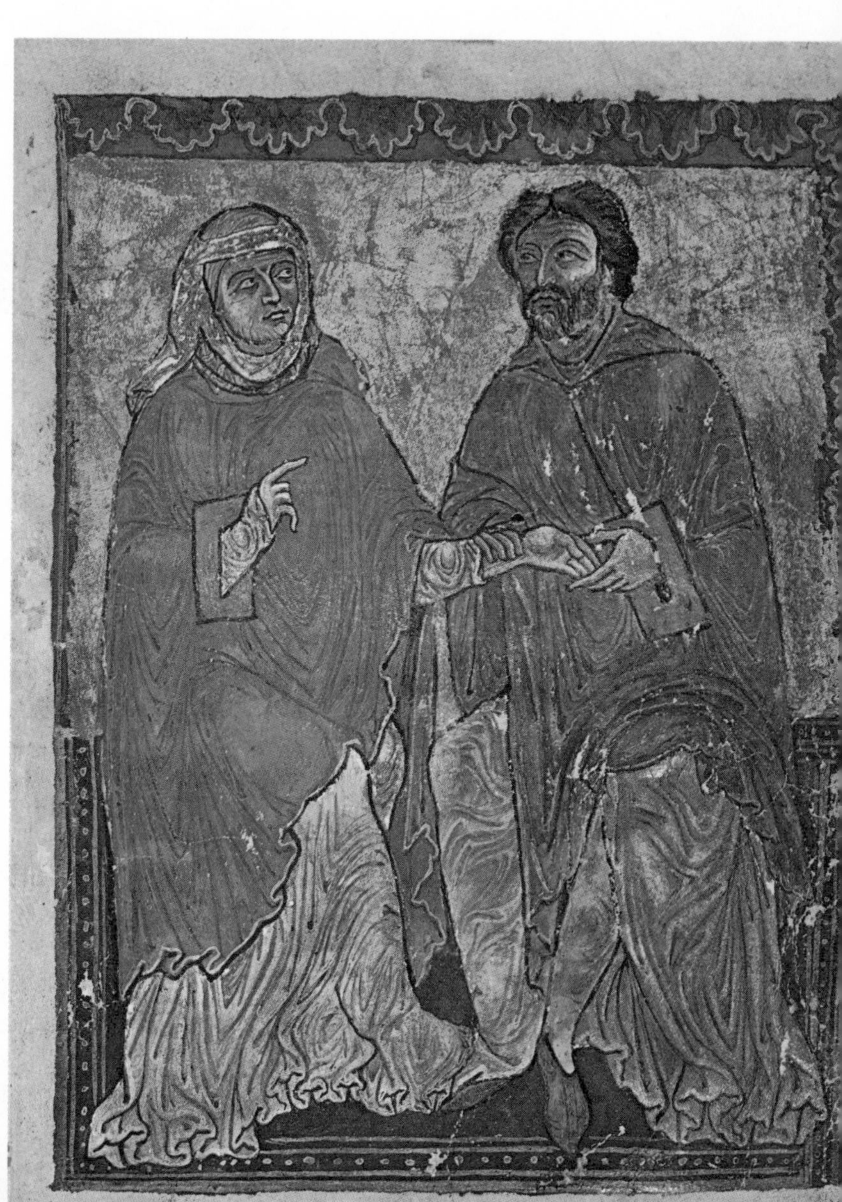

world, wrote: 'How is it possible to believe that red-hot iron could lose its natural heat and grow cold for no adequate reason, or that because of a guilty conscience the element of water refuses to drown the accused?' The second event was the publication of Dante's treatise *De Monarchia*. This justified the existence of the State as the *natural* structure of man's political life. Dante believed that the right of the State to exist and govern did not emanate from the Church, but from a *law of nature,* according to which the social order depends upon government; and since the laws of nature express the will of God, the power of the State proceeds directly from God. To sum up: both in the cosmic and in the social order, things happen as *it is natural* for them to happen. This concept of 'naturalness' and thence of *physis* or *natura,* took firm hold of the medieval mind. It is hardly conceivable that writings such as those of Gregory of Tours and the *Life of St Nilus* could have been produced by an educated author of the thirteenth century.

How did medieval thinkers succeed in Christianising the *physis* and *technê* of the Greeks? In the same way that medieval physicians, a little later on, were to convert medicine into a true *ars medica?* In the same way that the pagan Galen became the inspiration and founder of the Christian art of healing from the thirteenth century onwards? In my opinion there were three decisive theological and cosmological concepts which enabled the Christian mentality of the Middle Ages to absorb Greek *physiologia:* that of God's 'ordered power', that of 'secondary causes' and that of 'conditioned necessity' or necessity *ex suppositione*.

God's power is infinite and absolute; God can do everything that is not in itself contradictory; but in the free use of his absolute power, it was God's will to create the world as it is. In regard to the existing state of the world, divine power is therefore 'ordered' (*potentia Dei ordinata*), and it follows that, except for the intervention of God's infinite power in some extraordinary and miraculous way in the world, stones can have no weight, nor fire heat.

This implies that in the causal processes of the universe there are two interconnected phases: the original and outstanding causality of the 'first cause' – namely God himself, who wished to create the world and to maintain its existence – and the subordinate causality of 'secondary causes', by means of which weight is a natural property of solid bodies and heat a property of fire. God created the world in such a way that solid bodies must have weight and fire must give heat. Stones are heavy and fires give heat 'from necessity', and thus the temporal disposition of secondary causes can be understood as being governed by a certain natural and immanent necessity in no way diminishing divine omnipotence, but rather resulting from it: this is destiny or *fatum* (as Aquinas expressly called it), the Christian form of the *anankê physeôs* of the Greeks.

'Necessity' may be interpreted in two ways, however. There is 'absolute necessity', such as that on which the heaviness of the stone and the heat of fire depend. As I said before, it is impossible for the stone to be without weight, or for the fire to give no heat. And this indicates that there is another order of necessity – 'conditioned necessity' or necessity *ex suppositione*.

A horse's white colour is not part of its specific nature, for there are also black and sorrel horses. But neither are we entitled to say that the actual whiteness of an individual horse has come to pass *ex suppositione.* To God, everything in the world is necessary *ex suppositione:* His creations exist and are as they are because He willed it so; the divine will and intelligence are the *suppositio* of the ordered and providential necessity of the *fatum.* For man, on the other hand, the reality of the created world and certain qualities of that reality – the heaviness of stone or the heat of fire – are absolutely necessary; whereas others – such as the habit of eating a certain sort of food, and the biological results of this diet – are only necessary *ex suppositione;* and this means that they may be controlled by man's will and intelligence – or more explicitly by his technical skill or 'art'.

This brief summary enables us to understand how the Greek notion of *physiologia* was absorbed without difficulty into the medieval mentality. We will take an example illustrating the subject with which we are concerned: the *technê iatrikê* or *ars medica.*

The art of healing involves a remedy, a disease and a doctor. Why do remedies cure? Because God wishes them to: 'Every cure proceeds from the ultimate good' (*omnis medela procedit a summo bono*) said Arnaldus de Vilanova at the end of the thirteenth century. But in fact God wished his absolute power to cause remedies to cure by being what they are – by virtue of their natural properties. The statement that an opiate causes sleep because it naturally possesses *dormitive virtue* is of course scientifically unsatisfactory, as Molière's genius made

Bringing the host to the sick. Archimateus of Salerno advised a doctor to ensure before starting treatment that his patient had confessed. From a fourteenth-century English manuscript.

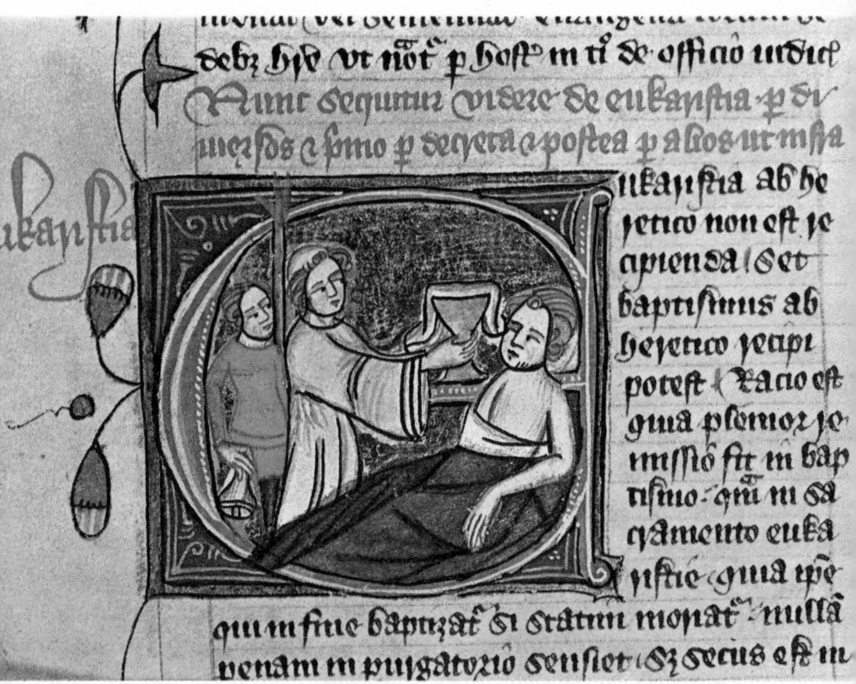

clear to everyone; but it remains for all that a fundamental assertion. Thus we see Greek doctrines of pharmacy incorporated in the thinking of the Christian West.

It is the same with illness. The development and course of an illness is usually no more than conditionally necessary to man (*ex suppositione*), and this is the reason why it can be avoided or cured by medical skill. Does this mean that *all* illnesses belong to the category of conditional necessity? As the heir to Greek thought, medieval Christianity – whether medical or no – saw an element of absolute necessity in man's illness. Falling ill is a permanent possibility: it is part of man's nature that he may become ill at any moment. Moreover certain definite ways of falling ill – certain diseases – appear to be subject to absolute necessity both in their onset and their development. To the *fatum* of human nature, a man of the Middle Ages would say, there mysteriously and 'necessarily' belongs the existence of mortal and incurable diseases, and the physician's art is powerless to deal with them. The Italian humanist Coluccio Salutati expressed this very clearly in the last years of the fourteenth century: 'It must be recognised that medicine is only useful and necessary in the case of curable illness. Or, to be more exact, that there is only need for medicine in those illnesses that nature could with difficulty conquer unaided.' Salutati's thought is crystal clear. Like all the men of his time, and like the Greeks before him, this humanist of the end of the Middle Ages distinguished three categories of illness: those that were cured by nature alone, those that required the help of the doctor's art, and those beyond its reach, because they were 'of necessity' mortal or incurable. The Greek notion of *anankê physeôs* thus persisted in medieval pathology and philosophy.

What sort of doctors were the physicians of this period? Just as a Hippocratic Asclepiad was the 'servant of nature', a Christian Galenist was the 'servant of God's ordained power'; the former adhered to his *logos,* the latter to his *ratio*. According to Aquinas, the internal source of healing was the 'virtue of nature' – and therefore the *ordinatio* of divine power, and its external source was the physician's art; art imitates nature and can do no more than help her. This is equivalent to saying that the possibilities of the art – 'the true reason for those things which *can* be *done*' according to the well-known scholastic definition – are limited by laws of nature whose necessity is absolute and not conditional. Thus, using his rational powers and within the limits imposed by the divine ordination of nature, a doctor invents or learns his art, and uses it to help cure the sick. The *technê iatrikê* of Hippocrates and Galen thus becomes converted into the *ars medica* of Christian Galenism, which was to rule medieval and Renaissance Europe from Taddeo Alderotti to Jean Fernel and Luis Mercado.

But let us return to our problem: the philia of doctor for patient in the 'technical' period of medieval medicine. After the central decades of the thirteenth century, in what way did the doctor express his philia for his patient through his art, and his love of it?

According to the Christian interpretation of human love, it should have as its special object the good and perfection of the soul of the beloved. On the other hand, love of one's art has as its immediate object the perfection of *nature* that may be achieved through it – i.e. the curing of the sick, in the case of the physician's art. The essence of our problem is, therefore, clear. In ideal circumstances, how could a medieval Galenist combine 'love for an individual' – the patient in this case – with 'love of his art' in 'technical philia' for his patient? Medieval technical medicine solved this problem in the only

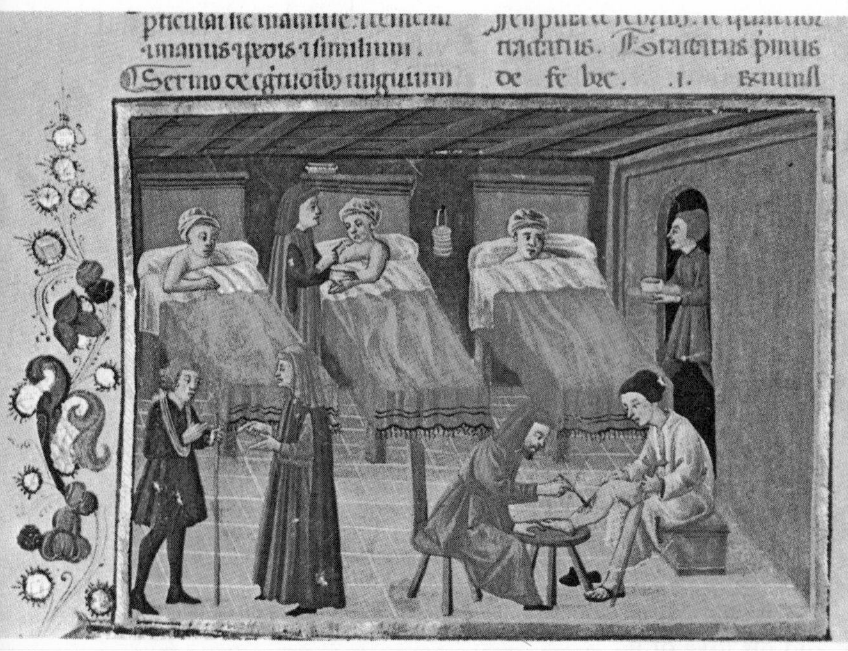

A three-bed hospital of the fifteenth century.

possible way, by a Greek interpretation of Christian thought: it simply combined the behaviour derived from 'Christian love of man' (consoling the patient and paying attention to his spiritual welfare) with that derived from 'Christian love of the doctor's art' (diagnosis and treatment, by which he co-operated with the 'ordained power' of God). And the former behaviour contributes to the effectiveness of the latter.

A careful reading of what was written about the pathology and rules of medical policy after the first half of the thirteenth

Medical care in the home. From a Flemish manuscript. Gentlewomen administer to the daughter of the prince of Salerne, who has poisoned herself for love.

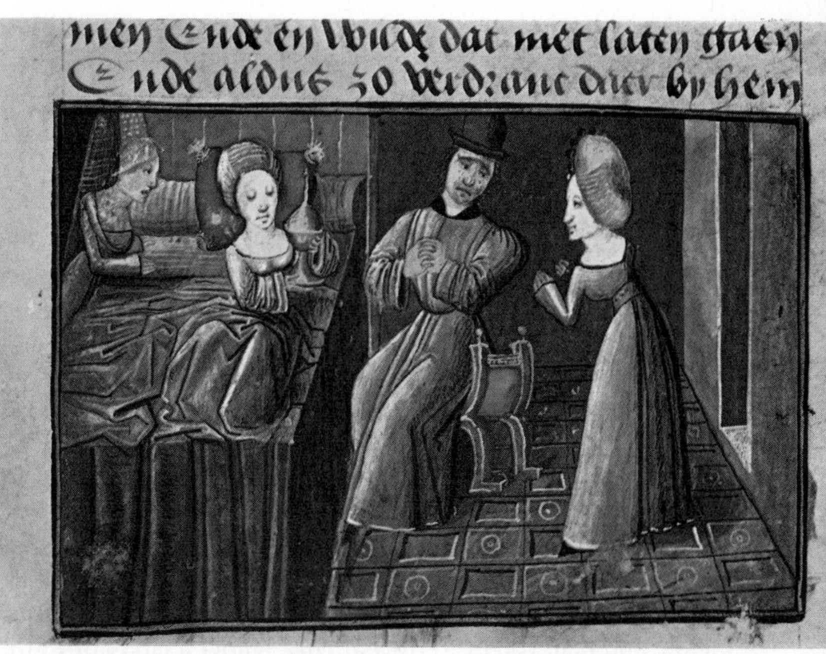

century makes this clear. The writings of Guglielmo de Saliceto from Piacenza and the Spanish doctor Arnaldus de Vilanova are outstanding. In his *Summa conservationis et curationis*, Saliceto tells the physician what his relation to the sick man and those who summoned him should be. If he takes his pulse with a serious and attentive air he will gain the confidence of both, 'and this is of immeasurable use in good medical practice'. With subtle psychological and clinical intuition, our author sees that the way the patient is questioned can be therapeutically valuable: 'The sick man's spirits are comforted thereby . . . and the remedies have a more marked action . . .; the invalid's spirits are so fortified by virtue of this faith and imagination as to affect the malady more intensely, freely and delicately than the doctor himself with his instruments and medicine.' The advice given by the surgeon from Piacenza about the physician's relation to his colleagues and those who know nothing of medicine is equally penetrating and careful. The precepts of Arnaldus de Vilanova in his *Cautelae medicorum* are more rhetorical and high toned, and perhaps show a greater awareness of the doctor's dignity: 'The physician should be studious as to learning, careful and methodical in prescription, judicious and prudent in his replies, ambiguous in prognosis, true to his promises; and he should not promise health, for in so doing he will usurp the divine office and cause offence to God. Rather must he promise fidelity and diligence; and he must be discreet in visiting, ready in discourse, honest in his sentiments, and benevolent to the patient.' Under a cloak of Latin and Christianity, the tone and feeling of the Hippocratic *Praecepta* is reborn.

But was the medieval doctor's love for his patients always so perfect?

Medicine and the society of the Middle Ages

Without going into minute details of the diagnosis and treatment of the period, I must briefly explain how the juxtaposition of 'love of man' and 'love of art' was achieved.

The medieval physician's behaviour was not, in point of fact, a belated Latin copy of that of his masters in the art of healing – Galen and Soranus in classical Greece, Ali Abbas and Avicenna in Asiatic Islam. Influenced by his Christian conscience, by concern for his professional reputation, or – as we shall see – by the stern dictates of the law, the medieval healer was well aware of his patient's personal status and the religious duties belonging to it. Naturally these were strictly un-technical, and unless the doctor was also a member of the clergy, they must be attended to by a priest. The 'natural character' (*individuatio naturalis*) of the treatment was exclusively technical and followed the rules of the Graeco-Arab *ars medica*; on the other hand the 'personal or spiritual character' (*individuatio personalis sive spiritualis*) of helping the sick man was almost exclusively a moral and religious matter.

Almost exclusively. As I have said before, the medieval doctor tried to give some internal unity to this simple juxtaposition. From his own experience – for I do not think that Plato's *Charmides* or *Laws* had much influence on medieval physicians – he had discovered the value of talking to the invalid. The extract from Saliceto is relevant here. This helped the clinician to adapt his treatment to individual patients more effectively and coherently than he could by simply combining Galenic 'indication' (*endeixis*) with Christian piety. This was as far as he went, however, and the task of technically individualising the inevitable naturalism of medicine was not undertaken until our own century.

A sick man is not an isolated individual, however, but a member of the society to which he belongs – in this case,

A clinic, possibly the hospital of a medieval borough, from the French manuscript *De Proprietatibus Rerum* by Bartholomaeus Anglicus.

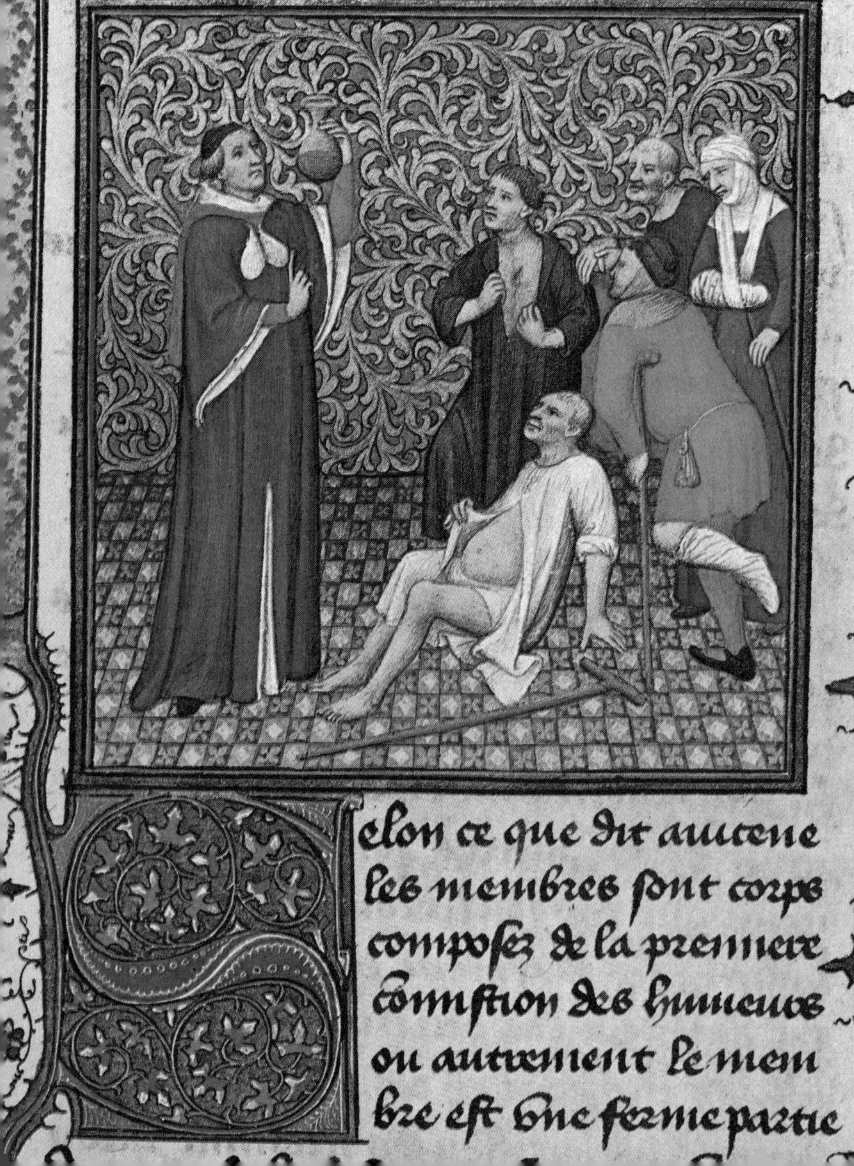

medieval society. We have seen what sort of treatment was provided in the monasteries of the Middle Ages. Medieval society was still feudal in country places, but incipiently urbanised in the towns; what would happen when it developed a coherent structure? How would this new world give social expression to the case of the sick? Basically, in the following two ways:

First, by making laws to regulate the different aspects – economical, religious, moral and political – of the links between medical practice and society. Faithful to a constant principle in the history of western culture, medieval society admitted 'medical philia' in theory, while at the same time mistrusting it sufficiently to subject it to the authority of written law.

Secondly, by establishing definite social distinctions in the treatment of the sick. The threefold classification we found in ancient Athens persisted, *mutatis mutandis,* in the intensely Christian society of medieval Europe. Arnaldus de Vilanova openly distinguished between 'medicine for the rich' and 'medicine for the poor'. This realistic attitude could be further elaborated by saying that it is possible to detect three separate levels of medical care in the latter part of the Middle Ages:

1 The 'poorer class', whether actual slaves, workers on the land, or poor townsmen. Medical care for all these was provided in hospital – one of the hospitals of the medieval boroughs, where every sort of nuisance, particularly smells, permanently prevailed.

2 The class of artisans and rising bourgeoisie. These were mostly cared for at home. The 'family doctor' began to make an appearance in the cities of the later medieval period.
3 The influential classes: princes, feudal lords, magnates of the Church. These patients were visited at home by a leading doctor, or one exclusively devoted to them, the *medicus a cubiculo*.

This organisation of medical treatment was a typical instance of the structure of medieval society.

The doctor's duties

Medieval society interpreted the relation between doctor and patient in Christian terms. A medieval version of Christian morality gave substance and shape to the ethico-religious aspect of the relationship. And since the notion of 'duty' is a basic one in all morality, let us see what were the chief obligations of a doctor to his patient.

Religious duties came first of all. A physician was morally and socially obliged to care for his patients and procure their bodily and spiritual welfare. In Spain, medieval laws regulated the most important religious duty of the doctor precisely: when a patient's life was in danger he must advise him to confess his sins. 'That the sick man must think of his soul before medicine for his body; and what punishment is deserved by a physician who treats him in any other way' is the heading of one of the laws of the *Primera Partida*. When a doctor visits a sick man, his first duty is to make him think of his soul, and confess. 'After this is done, the doctor must minister to his body, but not before: for it often happens that maladies increase and grow worse as a result of a man's sins.' The patient's bad conscience may aggravate the disease. And if the physician does otherwise, 'Holy Church would think fit to cast him out, for having acted against her laws.'

When the state grew more powerful, civil punishment was substituted for punishment by the Church. If a doctor paid two visits to a desperately sick man without persuading him to confess – so says a decree issued by Ferdinand and Isabella – he must pay a fine of ten thousand maravedis. This was a foreseeable consequence of the confusion between religious and political issues. Religious duty became a political duty, and prison or fines sometimes took the place of repentance, to the detriment of the freedom inherent in religious observance.

The *civil duties* of the medieval doctor were numerous. For instance, a very curious conflict was set up between the law (which tried to establish some uniformity in doctor's fees), and the interests of the physician himself, (who always aspired to the highest possible reward). Frederick II's decree of 1231, already referred to, is quite explicit in this respect. 'The doctor will swear ... to give free help to the poor; he will visit a sick man at least twice a day, and if it is required of him every night as well; and for this he will not receive more than half a *tarreno* in gold, unless he has been obliged to go outside the city or the camp.' Medieval doctors accepted their Christian obligation to give free treatment to the poor with a good grace. But why should a patient who was rolling in money pay a fixed sum? Surely the profession of doctor was a sufficiently onerous one? 'It would not be a bad thing,' wrote Saliceto, expressing the general view, 'to ask the highest possible fees for medical treatment, giving the examination of excrement and urine as a reason.' Lanfranc, another surgeon of the second half of the thirteenth century, gave even cruder and more summary advice: 'A doctor helps the poor when he can, but he is not afraid to ask good fees from the rich.' Western life has changed very little in certain particulars since the time of the Greek city-states.

The civil authorities of the Middle Ages framed rules that regulated many of a doctor's activities: medico-legal provisos, rules concerning hygiene, medical responsibility, fees, the preparation and price of medicines, and so forth. Society and the state were exerting more and more influence over the relation between doctor and patient.

3 The nineteenth century

The most important religious development in modern history since the Reformation has certainly been the progressive secularisation of western society and culture. There are and have always been many individual Christians in the West; but since the end of the eighteenth century, society itself has no longer called itself Christian; it has become secularised.

I am here using the word 'secularisation' to describe the historical experiences of modern western man, when he began to want to earn his living exclusively from the potentialities and resources inherent in his own nature – from his own reason, imagination and will-power. In other words: he wanted to eliminate anything that could be described as 'supernatural' or as 'revelation' from his historical development.

The process of secularisation began at the end of the seventeenth century and made rapid progress during the eighteenth and nineteenth. The history of its successive stages is well known. A freethinker to begin with, secularised man became a deist or a materialist in the eighteenth century, and a positivist, an agnostic, an anarchist or a Marxist in the two following centuries. This trend began with the intellectuals of the aristocracy and upper middle classes; the masses did not become secularised until well into the nineteenth century.

Let us now consider our problem. The middle-class society of the latter half of the nineteenth century was made up of Catholic Christians, Protestant Christians and secularised men, living side by side; however it was the latter who gave the dominant tone to collective life. What was the attitude and behaviour to his patient of a doctor, considered solely as a *fils du siècle?*

Secularisation of the doctor's role

Within this secularised society one might find a doctor calling himself a Christian, who practised his profession with the object of making money alone; but if asked about his motives, he would probably feel obliged to reply hypocritically that his activity was nothing but a professional form of giving Christian aid to his neighbour. Of course he was paid for providing it; but that was because 'one must live', and also 'for the reputation of the medical profession'. Strategically disguised and idealised, his duties were based on the Christian version of the *philanthrôpia* of the ancients described in the last chapter. How would a definitely secularised doctor reply to the same question?

To answer accurately, we must make a distinction between ethically admirable methods of practising medicine from those that are less so.

1 Let us take the second half of the nineteenth century or the first decades of the twentieth. Medicine has become secularised, as the beliefs and behaviour of almost all physicians of the West go to show; some of them definitely declare that they do not consider themselves Christians, others that they are Christian as to their consciences and the situations limiting their lives, but that they practice medicine according to the 'customs of their time'. It is impossible to ignore the fact that many of them have an authentic sense of vocation towards their profession and are directed by a delicate but strict morality. Hundreds of real doctors will be found having

much in common with those literary archetypes of medical practice, Perez Galdós' Dr Golfin and Albert Camus' Dr Rieux. Such men show by the professional and economic implications of their medical practice that 'philanthropy' – the secularised form of a Christian's love for his neighbour, not a return to the *philanthrôpia* of pagan antiquity – is the human basis of the technical help they provide.

But two very different forms of this modern secularised philanthropy can be distinguished. First, there are doctors whose view of human life, at least insofar as it controls their conduct, holds firmly to the concept of man as an *individual.* Man is not merely a piece of cosmic reality, but natural reality endowed with intimacy and freedom, and capable of developing personality – in fact a combination in a single being of 'cosmic nature' and 'spirit', though the latter no longer has a Christian interpretation. We might take as a paradigm of this secularised notion of an individual Kant's idea of man – *homo phaenomenon* and *homo noumenon* contained within the concrete reality of an individual human being, together with the moral concept of man's *noumenon,* and the attribution of autonomous aims freely chosen and accepted as the personal or 'noumenal' centre of our moral life.

If man's existence is conceived thus, philanthropy can still be true *friendship,* the loving pursuit of the friend's good for his own sake. The secularised view of the relation of friendship lays definite emphasis on 'respect' for the friend's inner self. 'Man is sacred' (*res sacra homo*) said the ancients; 'each man is sacred' (*res sacra unusquisque homo*) says the modern personalist. But of course the mutual 'respect' of secularised

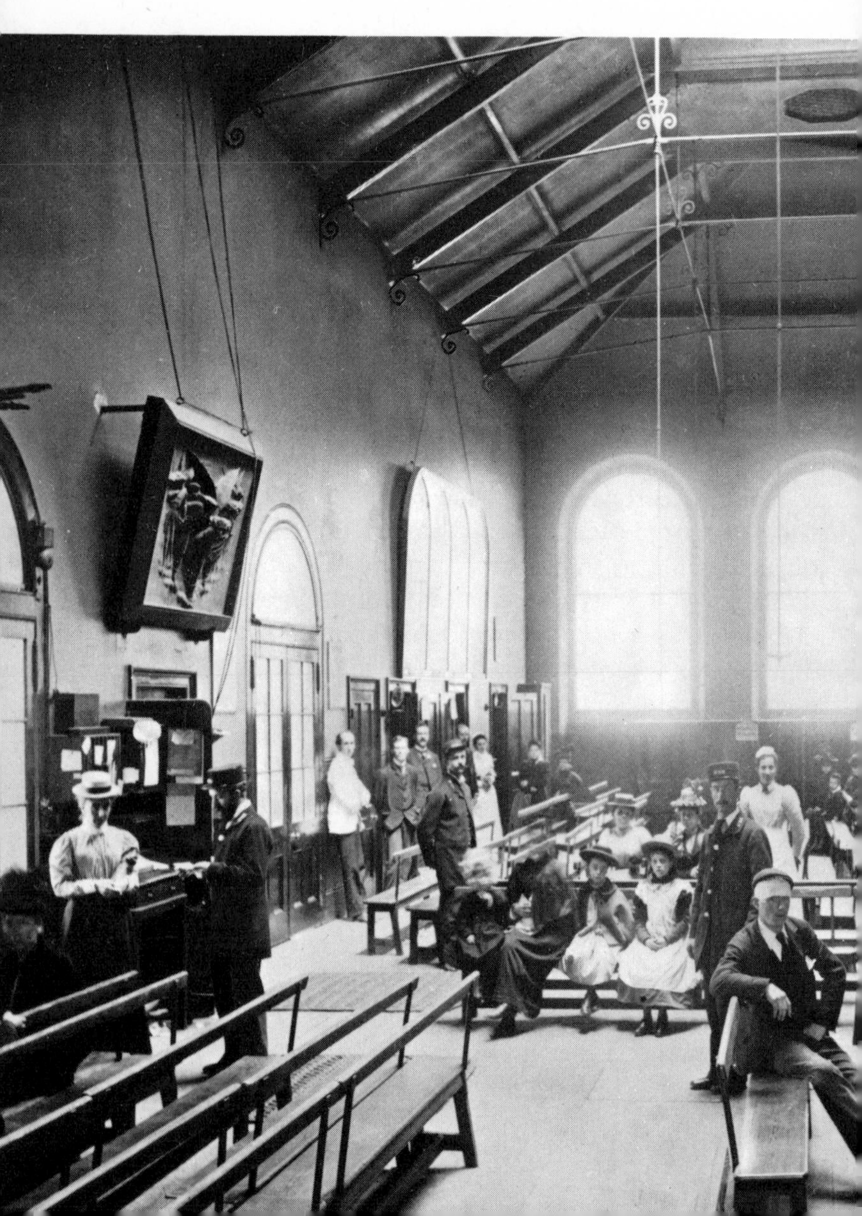

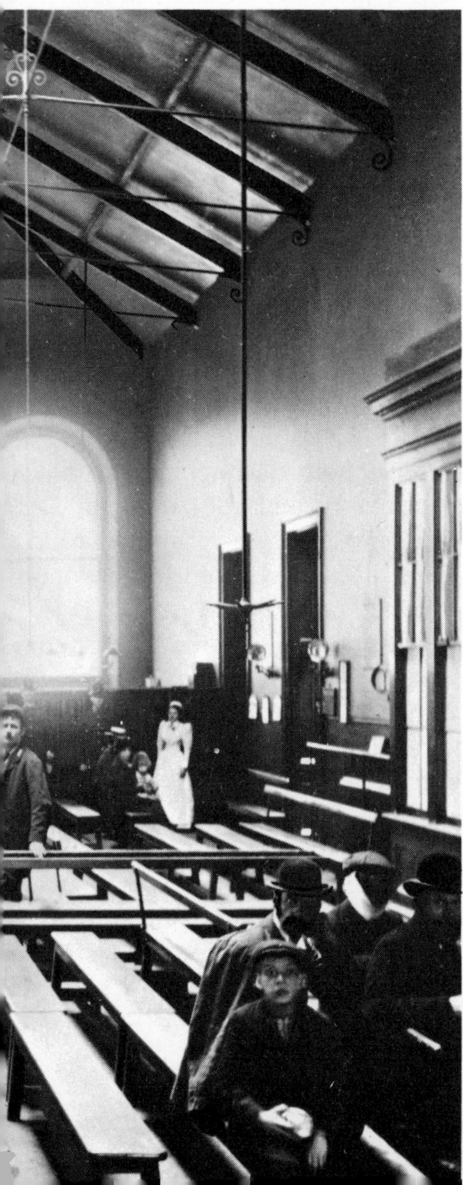

Outpatients,
at St Bartholomew's
Hospital, London,
probably *c.* 1904.
By this date there are
doctors who hold firmly
to the concept of man
as an individual
– a concept embracing
his 'cosmic nature' and
(in a de-Christianised
sense) his 'spirit'.

friendship – the *Achtung* of Kant's exquisite theory of friendship – is merely a secularised form of the Christian belief in the 'sacredness' of neighbours. According to this view, secularised friendship is a habit of human life, in which amiability, pursuit of the friend's welfare, confidence and respect are all combined.

Let us now see what becomes of benevolence in a man who has completely renounced the idea of the soul. All through the nineteenth century anthropology was developing along purely naturalistic lines, with man considered entirely and solely as a part of *the natural order*. There was no question of a return to the *physiologia* of the Greeks; the assumptions and forms of naturalism had undergone a radical change, and the champions of the scientific form of this new naturalism (Haeckel, Huxley, Lombroso, Vogt, Moleschott, Büchner and Oswald) as well as the leading advocates of dialectical materialism (Marx, Engels, Lenin) had come a long way from the old Greek 'physiologists'. Personality and the soul were simply names, mere logical constructs; or, as some said, 'epiphenomena'. But with such a concept of man, what becomes of love of human beings, or philanthropy?

Many modern doctors have been and still are 'naturalist' in theory and 'personalist' in practice. In practice, they desire and strive for the sick man's good for his own sake, and feel benevolence towards him as a fellow human-being, not because of the part he is playing in the world. But when anthropological naturalism is the result, philia ceases to exist and is transformed into *comradeship,* or an alliance for the purpose of attaining some public or private object. The phrase used by Diomed in the *Iliad* when he decides to seek a companion for his undertaking – 'two walking side by side' – is perhaps the most complete definition of comradeship. It does not aim at the comrade's good for his own sake, but only insofar as he cooperates in the conquest of the good aimed at by them both.

In the secularised view of human life, therefore, philanthropy can be either true philia or simple comradeship. The ethically most admirable forms of medical practice are based (as we shall show) on medical philia in the one case, and on medical comradeship in the other.

2 Other less noble ways of practising medicine are of course to be found in a secularised society. And this leads us to summarise the four main motives activating doctors in the modern world.

First, there is the doctor who, whether through philia or comradeship, is moved by sincere desire to give technical help to the patient who has come to him. The 'ego' in control of such a doctor's practice of his profession is one 'that helps' (*ego adiuvans*); and if his sense of vocation and his desire to help the sick man are deep and consistent, he will not treat him ultimately or definitively as an 'object', but his medical relation will usually lead him to see him as a person in pain and in need of help.

There are other doctors whose chief aim is scientific knowledge and the power over nature it brings. In their case it is a 'cognitive ego', an *ego sapiens,* that confronts the patient and is eager to reach an objective and accurate diagnosis; once that is arrived at, they believe they should confine themselves to treating the patient with remedies of 'scientifically proved' efficacy. To them, the sick man is above all an object of rational understanding.

In the world of today, we more and more often find doctors working for state-controlled or independent institutions where the sick are cared for, and therefore as officials. The 'official ego' who contemplates and treats these patients might well be called the *ego fungens* (*fungor* = to carry out a function); and unless deeper and more personal interests intervene, he sees the patient above all as an active element of society, an effective part of the social machine.

Lastly, there are doctors whose prevailing concern is a more or less well dissimulated appetite for money and fame. We are reminded of the remark of Aristophanes' Chremylus: 'Where there is no reward there is no skill'. This doctor is dominated by an *ego cupiens,* and in his eyes the patient is above everything a source of gain. Most of the diatribes against doctors, from John of Salisbury to A. J. Cronin's *Citadel,* by way of Petrarch and Quevedo, are aimed at this unmistakable abuse of the art of healing.

It is hardly necessary to say that in every doctor two or three of these motives will nearly always be found intertwined, perhaps even all four of them, although one may dominate the rest. Doctors are not 'all of one piece': neither so inhuman that their sole object is scientific knowledge, service to the state or the opportunity to make money, nor yet so angelic that they practise medicine purely out of love of their art and the patient. For it to be morally permissible to practise medicine it is enough – given adequate technique –

Belief in remedies of 'scientifically proved' efficacy can go too far, as in Daumier's sad physician. 'How is it that, despite my store of drugs and purgatives, my patients all pass away?'.

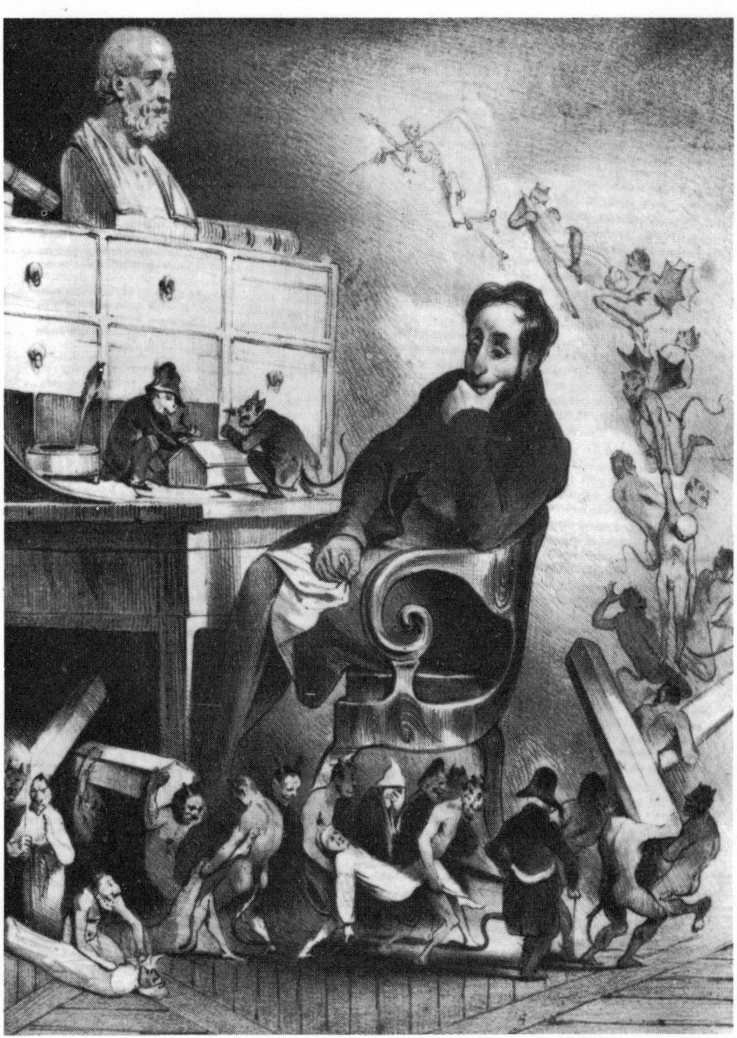

'The Undertakers' Arms', by Hogarth, a satire on inept and brutal quack-doctors. 'When an undertaker is in want of business, he cannot better apply than to some of those gentlemen, represented in deep consultation upon the contents of a urinal.'

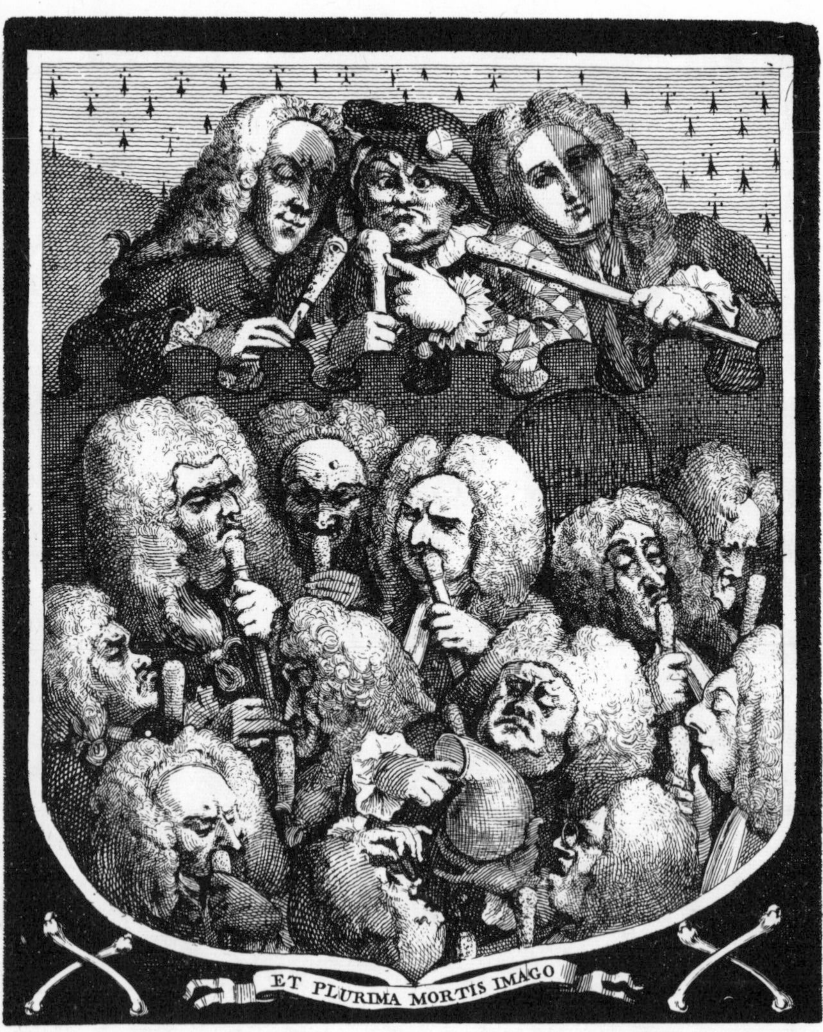

that greed for gain or prestige, or personal advantage, or a cold and inhuman appetite for knowledge should not decisively control the doctor's behaviour.

Let us suppose that one of these practitioners motivated only 'by filthy lucre' (*pro detestanda pecunia*) were asked what was the motive for his activity. What would he reply? Perhaps he would cynically admit the truth; but it is more likely that he would pretend that his intention was philanthropic. And thus we should get something resembling a secularisation – for vice too can be secularised – by which he disguised his far from secret greed for gain as Christian love of his neighbour.

3 Rather than embark on that moral underworld of medicine, let us keep exclusively to the nobler forms of professional behaviour, those in which the doctor's relation with the patient is based on philia or comradeship. What has happened in these cases to make the philia medical, or the comradeship therapeutic? The Greeks gave us the key: the doctor becomes the friend of his art by way of philanthropy, and the friend of the sick man – or his comrade – by way of his love of man and medicine. What we want, therefore, is to find out in what sense the modern secularised doctor is the friend of medicine – or a 'technophile'.

When belief in free will and nominalism was at its height during the later Middle Ages (Scotus, Ockham, Durand), a concept of natural science and technique – or 'art' – came into being which was very different from the one we saw established in the thirteenth century. Man showed that he was created in the image and likeness of God – such was the current belief –

not by his rational intelligence as Aquinas had affirmed, but by the freedom of his will, his liberty. The concept of the relationship between man and nature therefore changed; for if all natural 'necessities' were by the free will of God necessary *ex suppositione,* the same thing would be true in human terms in the case of man. Contrary to what the Greeks and the Hellenised Christians of the thirteenth century had believed, man's art, ability and technique in dealing with nature would in principle have no limits that could not be overcome. Thus there dawned in the minds of the men of the later Middle Ages an awareness that human power over natural 'necessity' or 'compulsion' was limitless – in fact the belief that constituted the central nerve of the 'modern outlook'. The technical Utopia described by Roger Bacon in his *Respublica Fidelium* was perhaps the first sign of this new attitude. And from that time up to the present day, the idea that what is impossible today will be possible tomorrow – the belief in the indefinite progress of technique – has ever more explicitly and vigorously controlled man's destiny.

A modern secularised physician's love of his own art is the result of the secularisation of this ambitious interpretation of the 'art of healing'. The doctor now sees his knowledge as being constantly added to by achievements that enable him to penetrate man's nature asymptotically and control it technically 'from above'; the Faustian spirit in modern man thus controls the will and mind of pathologist and therapist. Let us examine from this point of view the three ingredients that go to make up a medical event: the illness, the remedy, and the doctor himself.

With regard to illness, nineteenth- and twentieth-century medicine shows the increasing strength of the three following beliefs: first, no disease is 'necessarily' fatal or incurable; nothing in the disease can have *necessitas absoluta* for man. The sufferings that seem incurable today will be cured by the medicine of tomorrow. Secondly, the onset of disease is never 'necessary': in principle it can always be avoided. Thirdly, technical progress permits asymptotic penetration of the real nature of the morbid changes, both diagnostically and therapeutically.

As for the remedy, the inventions of modern therapy have followed in the path of Paracelsus, by way of the following stages:

(a) Artificial synthesis of the active principles contained in natural remedies: the use of chemistry as *imitatrice et rivale de la Nature,* to use Diderot's prophetic phrase.

(b) Artificial and synthetic production of curative substances that do not exist in nature and are more effective than any natural remedies (arseno-benzols, sulphonamides, etc.): chemistry no longer rivals nature, but surpasses her.

(c) Artificial modification – creative to some extent – of the patient's nature. Here is a significant paragraph by the biologist Jean Rostand: 'The prolongation of life, choice of a child's sex, posthumous impregnation, procreation without a father, test-tube pregnancy, pre-natal or post-natal modification of organic characteristics, chemical control of mood and character, genius or virtue to order ... all these now appear to us as desirable or possible achievements of the science of tomorrow.' The obvious irony in these lines should not make us overlook the deep and serious intellectual pathos that animates them.

All this goes to show that the *doctor* no longer sees himself simply as 'serving nature by means of his art', like the Hippocratic Asclepiads. Now he feels that he is the instructor, educator and sculptor of nature, in fact her lord and master, although in certain cases he may be forced to declare that his art is temporarily impotent.

If this account of a doctor's art since the middle of the nineteenth century is correct, what about his love of his art? At the present day, what combines with generic philanthropy to form the mainspring of a true medical vocation? It is surely the love of technical knowledge which controls and moulds nature and is ready for whatever the future still has in store, either in diagnosis or treatment. I shall return to this theme at the close of this book.

Medical practice

Let us now see how the doctor's attitude to his profession is socially realised, in the three main forms of medical care provided by secularised middle-class society: hospitals, general and private practice. Ever since classical Greece, the sick have been cared for on three separate social levels: the poor in hospital; the middle-classes at home or in the house of the family doctor; the upper classes at home or in the consulting-rooms of 'specialists' or medical magnates.

It is easy to imagine what the technical care of the sick must have been like in one of the famous nineteenth-century

Chemistry as 'imitatrice et rivale de la Nature': the chemist in his laboratory, 1829. (Nature, barely visible, is glimpsed outside the window.) From William Pope's *Triumphal Chariot of Friction.*

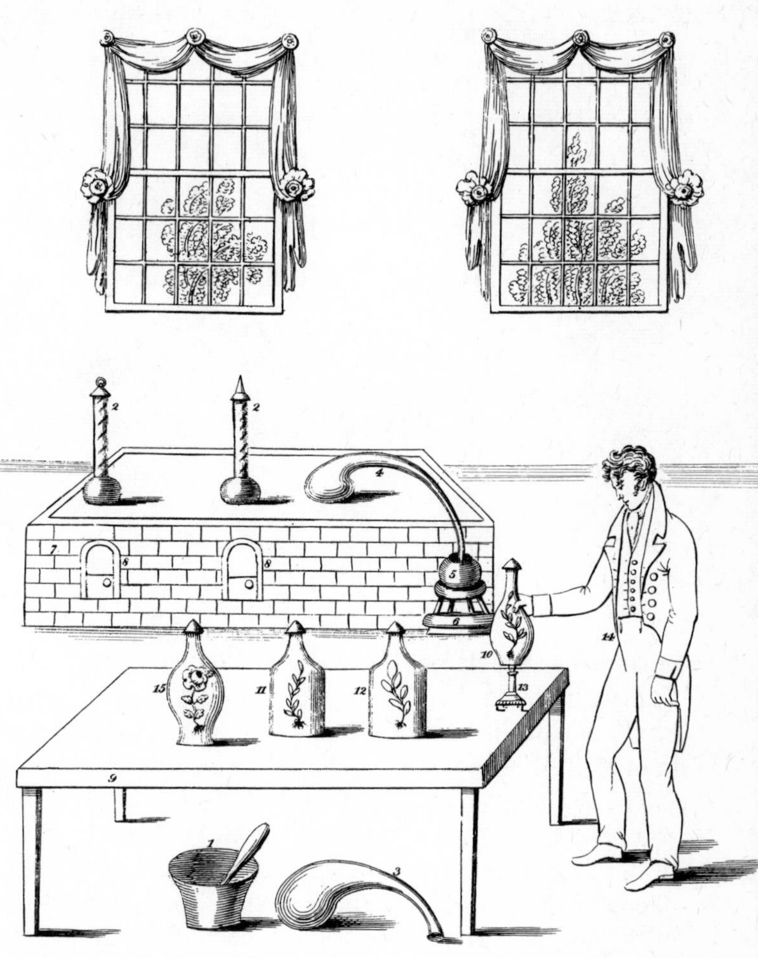

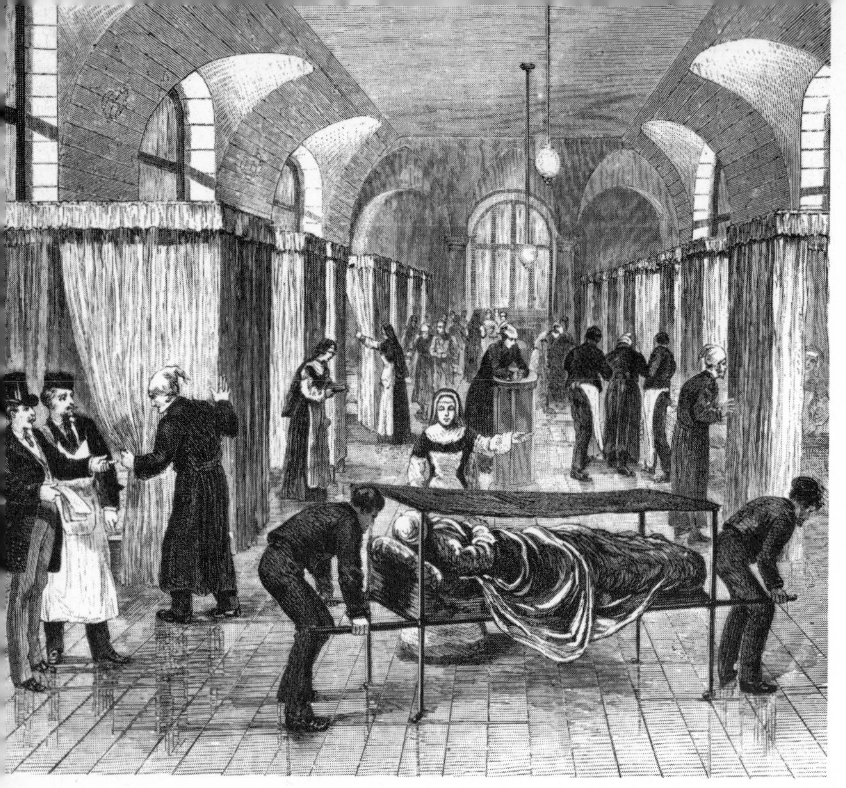

hospitals – the Hôtel-Dieu or the Salpêtrière in Paris, la Charité in Berlin, Guy's Hospital in London, the Allgemeines Krankenhaus in Vienna, San Carlos or the Hospital General in Madrid.

The patient usually arrived at the hospital in a state of mind combining confidence and resignation. He knew that, as part of his 'poor man's' treatment, he would receive an excellent diagnosis, because the hospital doctors were usually the best in the country; treatment, though necessarily limited by the never-abundant economic resources of the hospital; and finally a careful autopsy, if he should die. As the poor patients

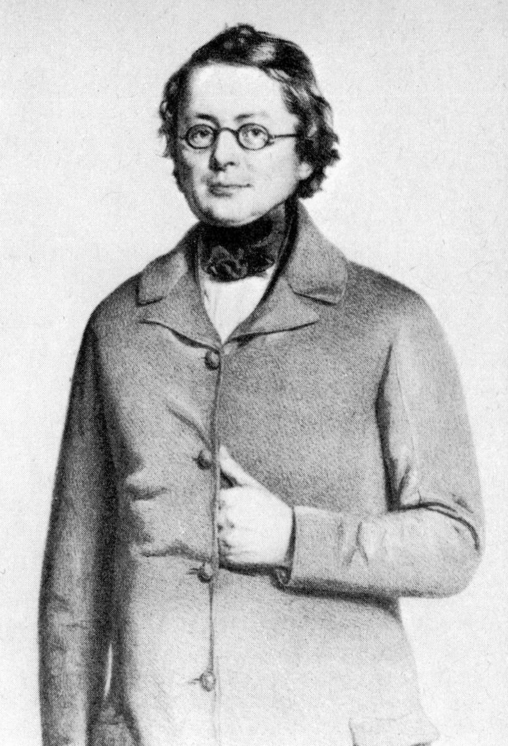

Left A ward in the Hôtel-Dieu hospital, Paris 1877.

Right Joseph Skoda (1805–81): his 'therapeutic nihilism' and over-riding concern for diagnosis put him at the opposite extreme from a doctor like Morton, or the Spanish professor San Martin.

of Vienna used to say ironically in about 1850: 'Viennese patients are lucky enough to receive an excellent diagnosis from Skoda, and an excellent autopsy from Rokitansky'. This belief was normally combined with a resigned and submissive attitude. The patient had more confidence in his doctor than in the hospital; he handed himself over with a wordless 'Here is my body, do what you like with it,' to the former, and 'See what an interesting disease I'm suffering from' to the latter.

How did the doctor generally respond to this attitude? Two types of hospital doctor of the nineteenth century must be distinguished; I will call them the *Skoda type* and the *San Martin type*.

The *Skoda type* is best illustrated by an anecdote about the hospital practice of the famous Viennese doctor. At the end of one of his spectacular diagnoses, Skoda failed to prescribe anything; and in reply to the assistant on duty, he replied: '*Ach, das ist ja alles eins!* (Oh, well, it makes no difference!)'. A similar tale is told of the great Addison, going his rounds in Guy's Hospital at about the same date. There were good reasons for Skoda's 'therapeutic nihilism' (Erna Lesky); it is enough to remember the state of medicinal resources in 1840. Skoda's clinical behaviour was not entirely nihilistic, but nevertheless two facts emerge: that his interest was unfailingly attracted to problems of physical diagnosis, and that he was lacking in that 'therapeutic enthusiasm' which made possible the feats of Paracelsus, Ambroise Paré, Withering, Morton and Jackson – an enthusiasm springing partly from an intense pleasure in manipulating and dominating nature, and partly from a strong desire to help the patient at all costs. For Skoda, as for many other physicians of similar mind, the hospital patient was both a scientifically cognisable and modifiable object and an unknown individual.

Rather than a 'doctor' in the strictest sense, a clinician like Skoda was a 'naturalist', a man who was attracted by the idea of gaining an objective and scientific knowledge of nature, and who aspired to be a 'sage', *savant* or *Gelehrte*. It is true that but for this outlook much of modern medicine would never have existed; but was there a darker side of the coin?

I am of course alluding to the melancholy conditions of life

An operation in Massachusetts General Hospital, October 1846, using ether for the first time. William Morton was the anaesthetist. This is probably a posed photograph, taken about the same time, as the actual patient was a young man.

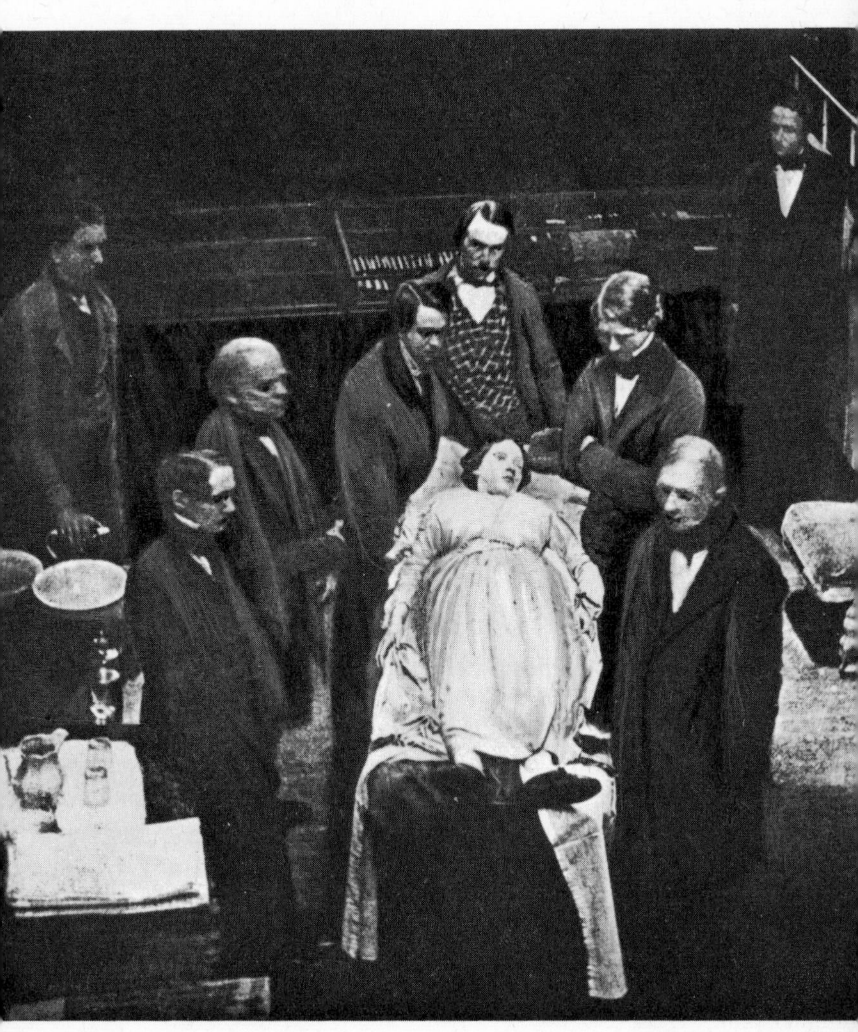

for hospital patients. We need only think of the daily scene in the surgeries of the Hôtel-Dieu in Paris, when the doctor on duty arrived every morning with a vinegar-soaked sponge held to his nose to avoid the terrible impact of the foul air in the room. But my previous question was mainly concerned with the effects of the doctor's attitude on his relation to his patients. Could it be a satisfactory one? If the doctor was an anatomo-clinical pathologist like Skoda, his true purpose and interests by-passed the patient himself and were focussed on his corpse – an imagined corpse when he diagnosed anatomical lesions *intra vitam* through physical tests (percussion, auscultation, etc.), and an actual corpse when this clinical diagnosis was confirmed or rectified on the dissecting table. It is not difficult to imagine how a patient felt towards a doctor from whom he could hope for nothing but a good diagnosis, followed by a good autopsy by the hospital prosector. Something of the same sort happened when the clinician's outlook was primarily physio-pathological. Then the doctor's purpose would be fulfilled in the laboratory. 'I consider the hospital merely as the vestibule to scientific medicine,' wrote Claude Bernard; 'as the preliminary field of observation into which the doctor must go; but the true sanctuary of medical science is the laboratory.' And many years later, remembering what life was like in a German hospital at the beginning of the twentieth century, Viktor von Weizsäcker wrote: 'A young assistant doctor's visits to the hospital did not last long, but his work in the laboratory took up hours and hours of day and night'. What the doctor was actually *observing* when he *looked at* a patient in the hospital ward was not his real physical and psychological condition, but the chymograph and retort awaiting him in the laboratory.

But not all nineteenth-century hospital doctors were like Skoda. There were others, possibly the majority, who belonged to the *San Martin type*. Alejandro San Martin was an eminent Madrid professor of surgery at the end of the nineteenth century. Going his rounds through the women's ward of the Hospital of San Carlos, he noticed that one of them – hardly more than a child – was weeping by herself on her bed; he went up to her and said gently: 'What are you crying for, my dear? Haven't you got anyone to cry for you?' A trifling thing: merely a few sensitive and sympathetic words, but they are enough to show that by the nineteenth and early twentieth centuries a man could be a hospital doctor and have a scientific-natural attitude to medicine, without being blind to the human and personal aspect of the poor invalid he was attending; he could in fact agree that a clinician should take the well-known advice 'always console' – *guérir parfois, soulager souvent, consoler toujours* – as something more than a fine phrase. To this sort of doctor, the patient was both a scientifically cognisable and modifiable object, and a suffering and pathetic individual. This in the light of present-day therapy, is certainly not a *desideratum,* but it is a good deal better than the 'divine rudeness' of Schönlein, or Skoda's sceptical aridity, or Addison's lack of interest in therapy. As the great doctor Gregorio Marañon said: 'A hospital patient must be treated as if he were a Knight of the Round Table.'

We must now take a look at the treatment given patients in their homes, and their relation with their 'family doctor'.

Nineteenth-century writers, like Balzac, Flaubert and Galdós, have left us sympathetic portraits of these humble heroes of the battle against disease. The family doctor knows the patient who has sent for him very well; he may even have known him since he was born. And the patient usually thinks of the doctor as 'a friend of the family'. So that in this case the doctor regards his patient both as a scientifically cognisable and modifiable object and a familiar friend. The exigencies of practice often force him to combine the two parts of this formula. No one has expressed this more clearly and eloquently than Claude Bernard: 'A doctor often finds that in his treatment of patients he must take into account what is known as the influence of the moral on the physical, and therefore a host of family or social considerations that have nothing to do with science.' But this passage of Bernard's not only states a factual truth; it also testifies to the limited knowledge of pathology possessed by this brilliant physiologist and by others of this period. Did the treatises on general pathology in use at the time on both sides of the Rhine, by the German Cohnheim and the Frenchman Bouchard, help doctors make a scientific connection between treating the patient as a 'cognisable object' and a 'well-known person and a friend'? Medical practice was becoming a skilled combination of 'true science' – pathology, learnt from books of the period – and kindly and acute 'common sense'. If anyone doubts this, let him read, in Freud's *On the History of the Psychoanalytic Movement,* the advice that the Viennese gynaecologist Chrobak declared, off the record, to be the most effective for treating hysterics.

Lastly let us consider medical treatment in the private consulting-room. An eminent physician – Charcot or Dieulafoy in France, Naunyn or Friedrich von Müller in Germany, Billroth or Nothnagel in Austria, Baccelli and Murri in Italy, Rubio or Madinaveita in Spain – is receiving in his own house the patients awaiting their turn in his waiting-room. Doctor and patient have never before met. What is the doctor's attitude to his patient?

There seem to me to be three chief possibilities. First, his dominant interest may be scientific; what counts for him, more than financial gain, is scientific knowledge of nature. For such a doctor, the patient is both a cognisable and modifiable object and an unknown individual. Secondly, his chief interest may be economic, the desire to make money. A good diagnosis is then of value as a means not to knowledge, but to financial gain, and the patient in this case appears both as a source of profit and an individual to whom he feels indifferent – although, since no one is inspired solely by greed of gain, he may later on form an extra-professional friendship with him. Thirdly, as well as scientific and economic interest, the doctor may posses a true sense of vocation. He will see his diagnosis both as a means to scientific knowledge and also as lighting the way to medical philia and therapeutic help; and even if financial reward is important it is not the decisive factor. To such a doctor the patient is both a source of profit and a friend to be pitied.

Hysteria as a temporary anatomical disorder: a woman reacting to stimuli while in a hypnotic trance. Photographs of a Charcot experiment at the Salpêtrière, expressive of a medical attitude that was to lead, after Freud, to the 'rebellion of the subject'.

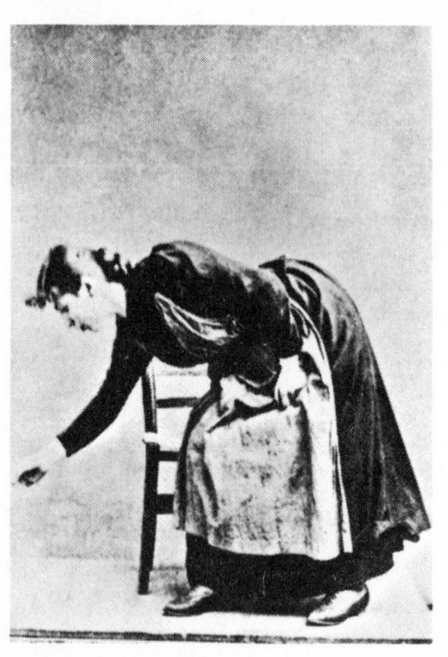

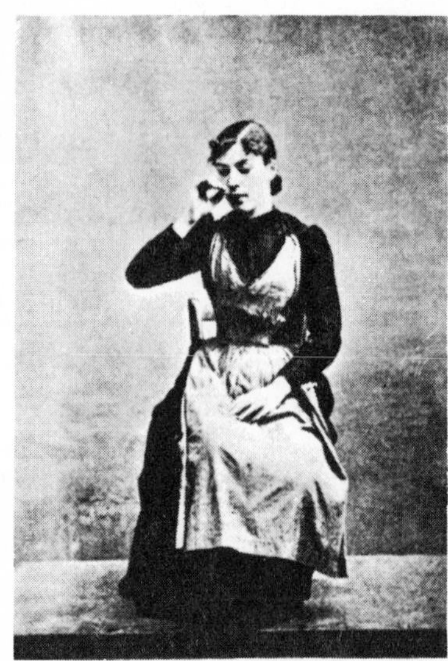

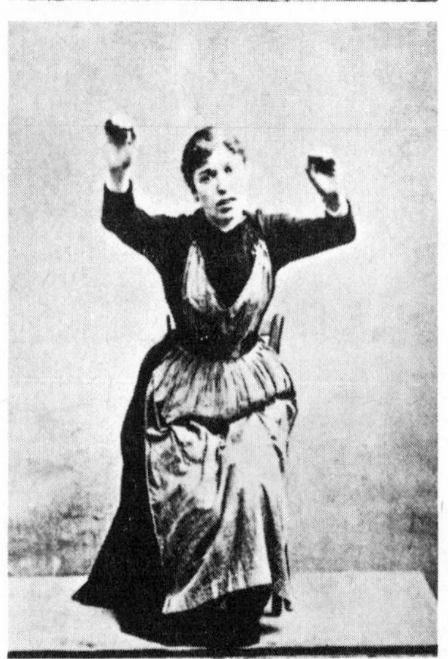

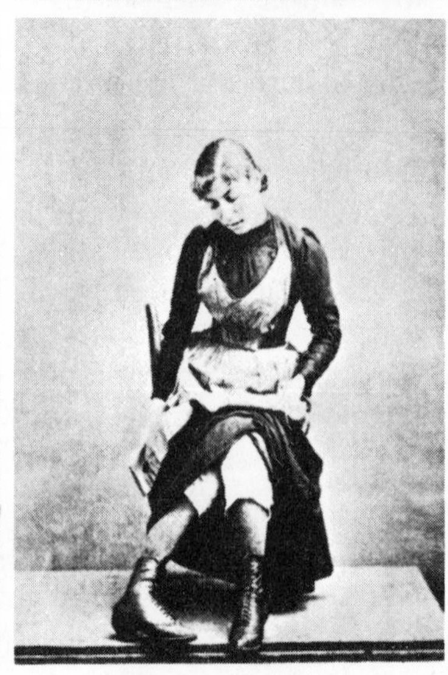

Crisis in medical care

Backed by a personalist view of anthropology – even though he may be no philosopher – the doctor by vocation realises his philanthropic feelings through 'medical philia', and uses his diagnostic and therapeutic abilities to procure the sick man's welfare and health. But if he entertains a scientific view of pathology, he will find himself – almost always unconsciously – dividing the patient into two scientifically disconnected halves: an 'object' (Kant's *homo phaenomenon*) and an 'individual' (Kant's *homo noumenon*). The social sphere in which this partition takes place – hospital, patient's home, or consulting-room – affects its psychological and sociological colour without altering it essentially.

The case is different when the therapist's view of anthropology is deliberately and definitely 'naturalistic', that is to say when his philanthropy is expressed in terms of 'medical comradeship'. Understood simply as correct natural functioning, the good of society or a means to the good of the state, health becomes an objective for doctor and patient to fight for together. But reality is more potent than doctrinaire theories, and man's reality insists that the doctor and the patient should be medical 'friends', not merely 'comrades' engaged in restoring the patient to health; so that the division between 'object' and 'individual' is in fact effected, under whatever name the patient may be classified. And whatever the patient's political and social ideology, can he really ever think of his *own* health merely as 'correct natural functioning', 'good of society' or 'means to the good of the state'?

There are two reasons – one clinical, the other social – why this attitude to the relation between doctor and patient became untenable. The former was the inevitable conflict between a pathology that reduced the patient to a mere 'natural object' and practice that stressed the importance of psychological and sociological data concerning the patient as an individual (see the passage from Claude Bernard already quoted). This conflict was particularly apparent in the illnesses that most clearly reveal the personal circumstances of the patient's life – the neuroses. How could the concept of hysteria as a temporary anatomical disorder (Charcot, Sollier), or as a functional change that could be studied through biochemistry or electrography (Empereur, Gilles de la Tourette, Cathelineau, Sticker, Riegel) solve the diagnostic and therapeutic problems of neurotic disturbance?[5]

But there were social reasons as well as clinical ones. The traditional distinction between 'medicine for the rich' and 'medicine for the poor' could no longer be tolerated, especially when, at the end of the nineteenth century and the beginning of the twentieth, therapeutic measures (such as drugs, surgery, etc.) became strikingly effective and notoriously expensive at the same time. Nor was this all. Besides receiving normal hospital treatment, patients had to lend their living bodies for clinical teaching purposes, and their corpses for the teaching of anatomy. As soon as a poor man fell ill, his body became *res publica,* or at least *res publicanda,* whereas the rich man's body was allowed inviolable privacy. For both clinical and social reasons, a crisis had been reached in the relation between doctor and patient.

The 'rebellion of the subject'

According to Von Weizsäcker, possibly the most deep-rooted and typical characteristic of present-day medicine is the 'introduction of the subject' into the physician's thinking and activity. The sick man is no longer a mere 'object' – even though he sometimes has to be studied objectively, he is now seen and treated as an individual. This is quite true. But it would not have been historically possible but for an earlier event, the 'rebellion of the subject', in which there is a social and also a clinical element. We will examine it in some detail.

The social aspects The great politico-social revolution of the modern world – exemplified by three dates: 1789, 1848, 1917 – can be noted to contain a more or less visible medical element. The origin of this profound revolutionary process lies in the general belief that has remained unchanged throughout its successive historical manifestations, that the political and social order prevailing in Europe since the early Middle Ages was neither just nor natural, but contrary to the dictates of justice, whether Christian or secularised, and to the laws of nature. As for 'human nature', it requires in itself a social order different from that of the *Ancien régime* and also from that of 'middle-class society', which supplanted the old stratified social order in the nineteenth century.

What was to be this new social order? How did it develop after the First World War? It is not the purpose of this book to answer these questions. I must confine myself to showing that this general and constant basis of Western social change

The conditions for life and work brought about by the Industrial Revolution were soon denounced by doctors. This detail from a map of Bethnal Green, London, shows the incidence of deaths from four classes of disease in a working-class area for the single year of 1838. The area shown extends for about half a mile. From Chadwick's Report of 1842.

involved a medical element, exclusively Western at first but very soon becoming world-wide: the rebellion of the individual against his own objective reality – his body – being treated unfairly and without consideration by the medical care available to him in the nineteenth and early twentieth century. In other and more concrete terms: the rebellion of the proletarian masses against the distinction between 'medicine for the rich' and 'medicine for the poor', and therefore against the relation to the patient implicit in the latter.

The facts of hospital life alone sufficiently justified the protest. For many years Spaniards spoke of 'hospital meat' to refer to those who could hope for nothing else but illness and despair. But perhaps a few sociological facts may be useful.

First of all the mortality figures. As soon as the industrialisation of the West began, a great difference was seen between the numbers of deaths in the industrial cities and in the rural parts of the country. C. Turner Thackrah, the pioneer of social medicine, over a century ago pointed out that in the industrial city of Leeds deaths were one out of every 55 people alive in 1821, whereas in a neighbouring country district the proportion was only one in seventy-four. 'At least 450 persons die annually in the borough of Leeds,' wrote Thackrah, 'from the injurious effects of manufactures, the crowded state of population, and the consequent bad habits of life that arise from it! . . . If we assume that 50,000 persons die every year in Great Britain as a result of injuries in factories, or as a result of their civil *status*, or the harsh conditions of some employment, I am sure that we shall underestimate the number.' This was

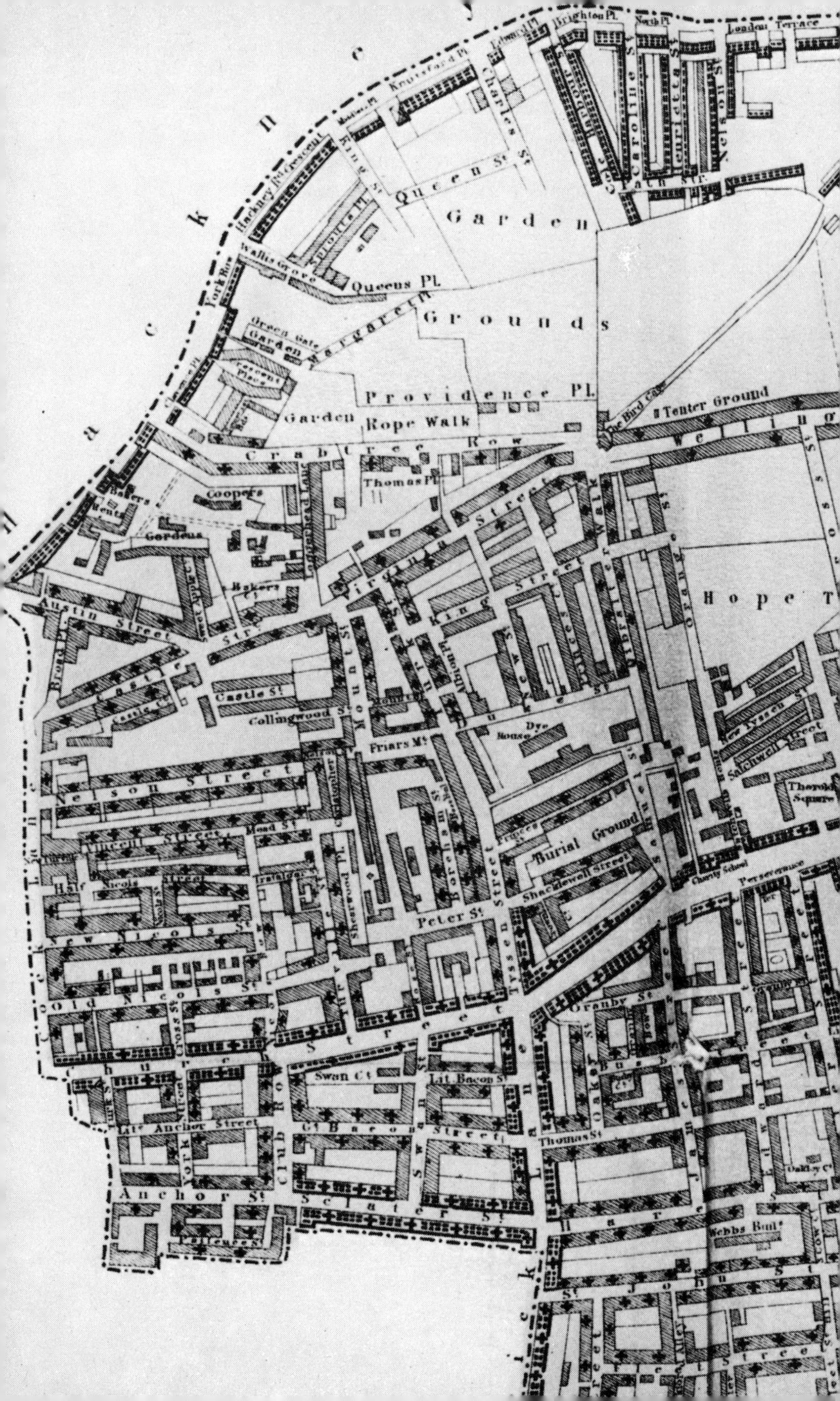
Brighton Pl.
North Pl.
London Terrace
Knutsford Pl.
Charles St
Hackney Rd. Crescent
Kings St
Queen St
Caroline St
Henrietta St
Nelson St
Garden
Walls Grove
Queens Pl.
Margaret
Grounds
Green Gate Garden
Crescent Place
Providence Pl.
Garden
Rope Walk
Tenter Ground
The Bird Cage
Crabtree Row
Thomas Pl.
Coopers
Gardens
Bakers Rents
Virginia Street
King Street
Hope T
Austin Street
Castle St
Castle St
Collingwood St
Friars Mt
Dye House
New Tyssen St
Satchwell Street
Nelson Street
Vincent Street
Burial Ground
Shacklewell Street
Charity School
Perseverance
Half Nicols Street
New Nicols St
Peter St
Tyssen Street
Old Nicols St
Granby St
Swan Ct
Lit. Bacon St
Gt Bacon Street
Thomas St
Lit. Anchor Street
York St
Club Row
Anchor St
Sclater St
Webbs Buil.
St John Street

Paracelsus' treatise on miners' diseases, 1567. This work is an earlier example of the social protest which doctors in the nineteenth century felt themselves more and more obliged to make. Statistics were the new conscience of the medical profession.

Theophraſti Paracel-
ſi von Hohenheim/ beyder Artzney Doctor ꝛc. Von der Bergſucht oder Bergkranck-
heiten drey Bücher / inn dreyzehen
Tractat verfaſt vnnd be-
ſchriben worden.

Darin̄en begryffen vom vrſprung vnd
herkom̄en derſelbigen kranckheiten/
ſampt jhren warhafftigen
Preſeruatiua vnnd
Curen.

Allen Ertz vnnd Bergleüten/ Schmeltzern/
Probierern/ Müntzmaiſtern/ Goldſchmiden/ vnnd
Alchimiſten/ auch allen denē ſo inn Metallen
vnd Mineralien arbayten/ hoch nutz-
lich / tröſtlich vnnd
notturfftig.

Mit Röm. Kay. Maieſt. freyheit.

Anno Dom̄ini 1567.

Leeds in 1821; not Manchester as seen by Marx and Engels a few decades later.

But let us come to our own century. In Paris between 1923 and 1926 the average number of deaths from tuberculosis was four times as large in the working-class district XIII as in the well-to-do district VIII. In a sector of district XIII containing seventeen blocks, with 4,290 houses and 185,000 inhabitants, the average death-rate rose to 480, six times higher than that in district VIII (R. Pierreville, 1936). No less eloquent are the statistics given by Rollo H. Britten for North America in 1934. In ten of the United States the figures of deaths from pulmonary tuberculosis per 100,000 persons between twenty-five and forty-four years old were as follows: 193·5 among unskilled labourers, 69 among skilled labourers, and 28·6 among the professional classes – seven times greater, that is to say, among the first than the last. Mortality in general was almost double – 13·1 as against 7. Finally, here are the results of the statistical research of Perrott and Collins into the medical and sanitary aspects of the economic depression of 1930:

1 The average number of cases of incapacitating disease was 48 per cent greater in families all of whose members were unemployed.

2 Among well-off families, now so poor as to need help, the figure for incapacitating disease was 73 per cent higher than in families whose economic situation remained good throughout the four years of the depression.

3 Among well-off families who had become slightly poorer, the figure for incapacitating disease was 10 per cent higher

Cottages and their cesspool at Preston, Lancashire, 1884. From a contemporary report.

than in families whose economic situation remained good.
4 In moderately well-off families that had become poorer during the depression the figure for incapacitating disease was only 17 per cent higher than in families whose economic situation had remained tolerable.
5 The figure for such diseases in rich families declining into poverty was 9 per cent higher than in families that had always been poor.

The facts concerning the hours of work lost through illness are equally revealing. According to Pettenkofer, illness was causing the loss of 3,400,000 days of work a year in Bavaria in the year 1873. In New York, sixty years later, illness caused the loss of 10,000 million dollars a year. What must the loss of a day's work have meant to a European working-man of 1873 in terms of every sort of privation? And who would suffer the most vital and direct damage as a result of economic collapse in New York?

Of course things became especially serious when disease developed into an epidemic and a violent and calamitous social scourge. Pilar Faus (in collaboration with José Maria López-Piñero and Luis Garcia Ballester, *Medicina y Sociedad en la España del Siglo* XIX. Madrid 1966) has studied in great detail the social consequences of the cholera epidemic of 1885 in the province of Valencia, and drawn highly revealing conclusions.

It must be emphasised that doctors themselves have been in the forefront of these denunciations and protests. The treatises on occupational disease by Paracelsus (*Von der Bergsucht und anderen Bergkrankheiten*) and Ramazzini (*De morbis artificum*)

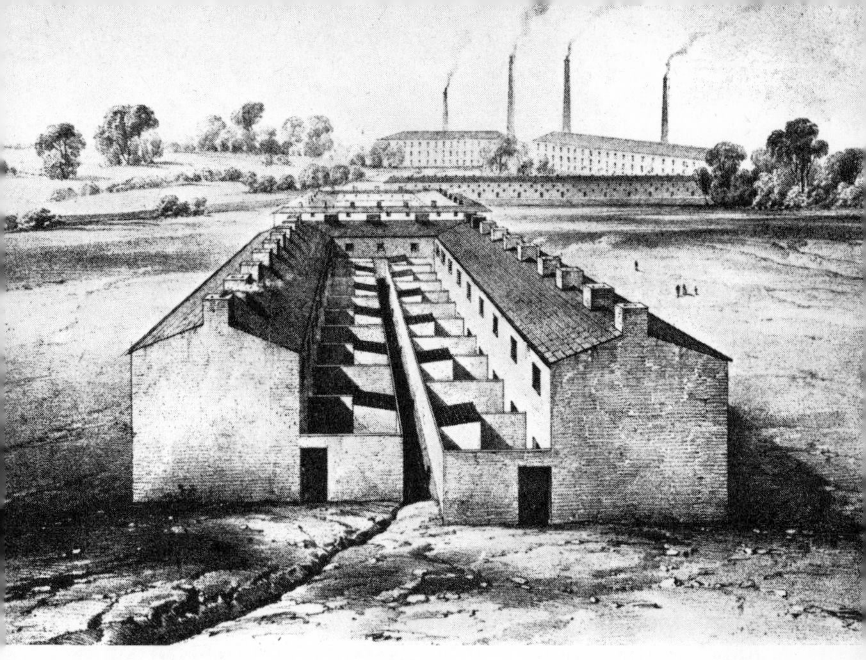

were more than mere clinical documents. But in the nineteenth century the doctors' protest became explicit and serious, and therefore socially significant. Industrialisation had made the differences between rich and poor greater and more obvious, and rapid developments in statistics provided a suitable instrument for studying them and presenting them accurately. I have already mentioned the work of Thackrah, soon afterwards amplified in the pages of E. Chadwick's monumental *Report on the Sanitary Condition of the Labouring Population of Great Britain* (1842). Rudolf Virchow's account of the sanitary conditions of the working-classes of Silesia in 1848 created great interest, both because the author subsequently became an eminent scientist, and because of the importance of the facts he described. The state of affairs denounced by the dramatist Hauptmann in one of his famous plays, had already been revealed fifty years earlier by Virchow. Villermé's report on the state of workers in the French textile industry dates from 1840. An excellent study by J. M. Lopez-Piñero has made known the honourable part played by Spanish physicians in this admirable joint enterprise of European doctors, some (like López de Arévalo, Masdevall and Ximénez de Lorite) during the eighteenth century, others (like Ruiz de Luzuriago, Seoane and Monlau) during the nineteenth.

The first reaction of the middle classes to this denunciation by the doctors could have been foretold. 'They believe, or profess to believe' wrote Thackrah, 'that the evils cannot be counteracted, and urge that an investigation of such evil can only produce pain and discontent'. However, it must be admitted that this was not the only way the bourgeoisie reacted, and that the sanitary and economic conditions of industrial workers started to improve steadily in Europe and America, about the middle of the nineteenth century. But we are not so much concerned here with the general history of these developments as with their effect on the relation between doctor and patient. Did some fundamental change in this relationship inevitably result?

Obviously the protagonists of this great social revolution – the working-class of the nineteenth and twentieth centuries – were not primarily interested in reforming the doctor-patient relationship. All they wanted was that, in case of illness, they should receive the same treatment as the rich: the same medicines, the same operating-theatres, the same facilities for investigation, better hospitals than were then available, compensation for accidents at work, and various forms of social insurance. But none of this was to be realised without an important change in the quality and basis of the medical relationship. In my opinion the principal elements in this change have been the following:

1 Instead of handing over his own body, with varying degrees of confidence, but unconditionally, the patient is now explicitly and effectively aware that he has a right to help when he presents himself to the doctor. From the first, the patient's relation with the therapist is based on the fact that he is 'entitled' to treatment. Medical assistance is therefore no longer mere hospital charity, and has manifestly acquired the character of a contract. The physician is no longer just a technician of healing, but also the nearest representative of 'society' – the impersonal entity responsible for providing assistance.

2 Where the doctor used normally only to be summoned in cases of serious illness, medical care is now in principle extended to all forms of suffering, including those that are slight or 'functional'.

3 Where the illness used to be endured and thought of as a disaster, it is now regarded also as entailing the advantages of free treatment or compensation.

4 Where the patient used automatically and unquestioningly to surrender his own body for clinical instruction, he now does so subject to conditions and vetoes. A patient's body has become his private possession, instead of *res publica*.

To sum up: the social element of the 'rebellion of the subject' has led to profound changes in the relation between hospital doctors and their patients. What form these changes have taken and what have been their results will soon emerge.

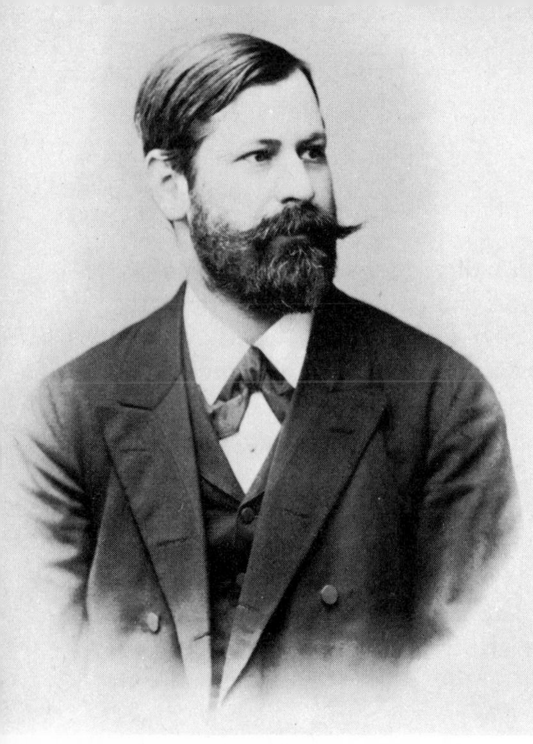

Sigmund Freud,
a photograph taken after
1901, when Freud was
in early middle age.

The clinical aspects Let us now examine the clinical aspect of the 'rebellion of the subject': the manner in which the patient has more or less consciously demanded to be clinically considered as an individual – or 'persona' – and not merely a useful or worthless 'object'. Social revolutionaries used to protest loudly and publicly against their ill-treatment. Nowadays rebellion takes a less violent and visible, but a subtler, form. The patient is in fact protesting against 'objectivation' itself, against the fact that, although he is an individual endowed with intelligence, intimate feelings and freedom, he is treated merely as an object now that he is ill.

Seen from this angle the patient's protest against objectivation has a name: it is *neurosis*. It seems that the frequency of neurotic phenomena has increased since the last decades of the nineteenth century, due, partly no doubt, to an increased tendency to classify problems under this title but also to historical and social factors, whose main ingredients I believe to have been two: on the one hand the greater demands habitually made on the somatic and psychic energy of the individual – in other words, social stress; and on the other to the crisis in the history of middle-class culture, incipient at this period – witness Marx, Nietzsche, Bergson, Strindberg and Unamuno for instance – and increasing to a notorious extent ever since. A man of the *belle époque* found himself subjected to increasing social stress, and he did not possess a stable system of historically-based beliefs which would enable him to survive it without psychic disorder. Are our current beliefs perhaps not such as to find satisfaction in effort and pain? The outbreaks of 'hysteria' in Paris and Vienna, the epidemic of 'colitis' so interestingly described by Axel Munthe in *The Story of San Michele,* Beard's 'neurasthenia' and Janet's 'psychasthenia', were some of the first clinical consequences of this state of things. But, as well as this diffuse historical and social cause, there was another strictly medical one affecting the obvious increase of neurotic phenomena during the transition between the nineteenth and twentieth century; this was the obvious inadequacy of traditional medicine, whether its chief orientation was anatamo-clinical, physio-pathological or bacteriological, to diagnose and cure this new and very important clinical development. If I may describe neurotic illness as 'rebellion', I propose to study this clinical aspect of the 'rebellion of the subject' in the case of hysteria.

Jean Charcot lecturing at the Salpêtrière. Freud called him one of the greatest of physicians, while recognising that their views on the nature of neurotic illness were irreconcilable.

In 1885 Freud, then a young Viennese neurologist, was awarded a grant to widen his field of research abroad, and decided to go to Paris, where he worked with Charcot. The latter was at the height of his fame, and was devoting his attention almost exclusively to the problem of hysteria. The wards of the Salpêtrière were full of hysterics, and though the newcomer's initial purpose was neurological research, Charcot's eminence, and daily contact with the theme of the moment, soon attracted him to it. His interest once engaged, would he follow the trail blazed by his master?

The publication of Freud's letters has enabled us to measure the admiration he felt for the demigod of the Salpêtrière. The qualified praise contained in his well-known obituary notice pales beside his spontaneous and frequent outpourings in his letters to his fiancée Martha Bernays. 'Charcot, who is one of the greatest of physicians and a man whose common sense borders on genius, is simply wrecking all my aims and opinions. I sometimes come out of his lectures as if from Notre Dame, with an entirely new idea about perfection', he wrote to Martha in November 1885. And three months later he confessed: 'Given favourable conditions I could achieve more than Nothnagel, to whom I consider myself superior, and might possibly reach the heights of Charcot himself'. Nothnagel was at that time the chief star of the Viennese medical firmament; yet the young Freud felt himself his superior. It was Charcot who seemed to be perfection, the almost unattainable goal to which this young man just under thirty might 'possibly' attain if circumstances favoured him.

But admiration does not stop at mere discipleship when the

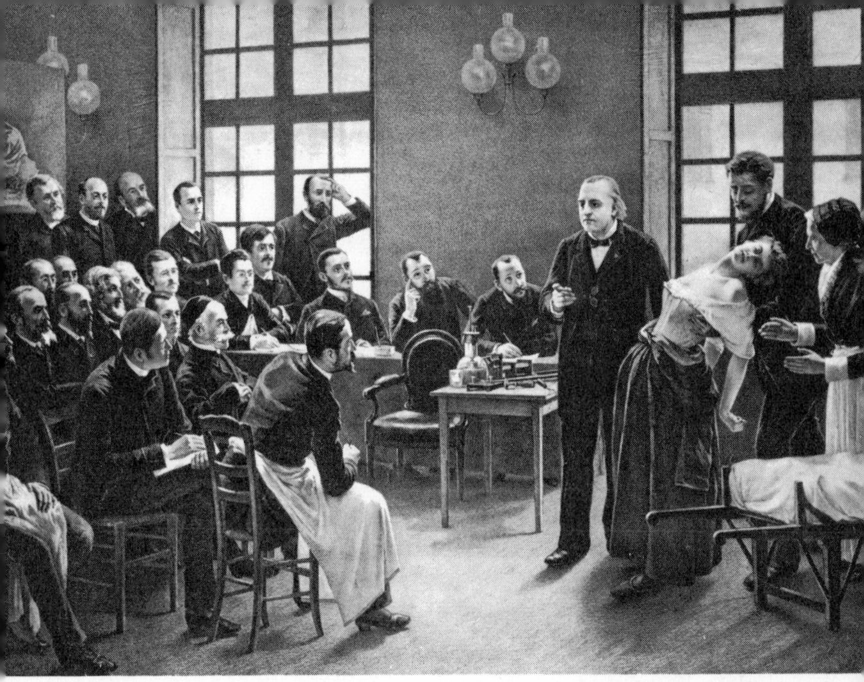

admirer is a man of genius. Charcot, whose powerful intellect was primarily visual – '*Je ne suis qu'un visuel'*, he used to tell his pupils – and whose medical training had been in the purest anatomo-clinical tradition, had just finished work on a theory of hysteria that was the product of his special gifts and his scientific training. Nosographically and pathogenetically, he treated hysteria, *mutatis mutandis,* as a morbid entity of the same nature as amyotrophic lateral sclerosis or *tabes dorsalis.* From the nosographic point of view Charcot saw 'major hysteria' as a clinical picture made up of a number of symptoms – convulsions, clonic spasms, *attitudes passionnelles,* deliria – that could be visually observed and were typically repeated in all patients. His account of them is like a series of film 'shots', identical for every patient. The disease of 'hysteria' was of the same order as the disease of 'pneumonia'.

Corresponding to this typical set of symptoms there must be a definite 'lesion', however brief, ephemeral and reversible, in the central nervous system. Charcot knew very well that an autopsy on the corpse of a hysteric could not reveal any visible anatomical lesions comparable to the easily seen traces left by amyotrophic lateral sclerosis or *tabes dorsalis*. But if a hysterical paraplegia reproduced the clinical picture of a spastic paraplegia caused by an organic spinal lesion, there were grounds for believing that some lesion had occurred in the spinal chord of the hysteric – temporary and capable of complete and immediate recovery, but none the less material and exquisitely localised – which was essentially comparable to what happened in an organic paraplegia. '*Au fond c'est le même syndrôme*', as Charcot wrote. The immediate cause of a hysterical disturbance would be a sensory-motor representation operating uncontrollably (*idée fixe*), localised in the nervous system, susceptible of being reproduced under hypnosis, and taking effect through the channels of movement and sensation described in anatomy-books. Symptomatology and pathogenesis combined to make hysteria, in spite of its apparent lack of anatomical lesions, a well-defined morbid anatamo-clinical condition.

This was not how Freud saw it. The first indication of his divergence from his master's doctrine, to be so clearly expressed later, was significantly revealed in a small event of 1886. Shortly before leaving Paris, Freud proposed to Charcot 'a plan for a comparative study of hysterical and organic paralyses'. His master listened kindly and attentively, but did not take up his pupil's subtle suggestion. 'It was easy to see,' Freud commented years later in his *Autobiographical Study,* 'that in reality he took no special interest in penetrating more deeply into the psychology of the neuroses'. And with great acuteness he added: 'When all is said and done, it was from pathological anatomy that his work had started.'

The significance of this slight but revealing difference of opinion is clear. As a research-worker and a clinician, Charcot studied *the* disease of hysteria and saw it as a real and typical psychosomatic disorder, whereas Freud preferred to study what the *patient's* hysteria meant to *him*, although he might not be fully conscious of it. For Charcot, hysterical paralyses must be localised in accordance with text-book anatomy, that is with the objective and permanent reality of the human body. For Freud, they were localised according to the idea the hysteric had of his own body. 'I wished to establish the thesis,' he wrote, 'that in hysteria paralyses and anaesthesias of the various parts of the body are demarcated according to the popular idea of their limits and not according to anatomical facts. The clinical picture of a hysteric would not therefore be determined by the *objective anatomy* taught by text-books, but by the *subjective anatomy,* as it were, always to be found tacitly present in the patient's mind, like some changeable and capricious form of popular science.

Two views of hysteria; two contrary methods of referring the hysterical symptom to the body of the individual who manifests or suffers it. Modern philosophical thought enables us to name them with all possible exactness. Charcot, the expert anatomo-pathologist, tried to account scientifically for hysteria in terms of the 'body from without' (Ortega), the

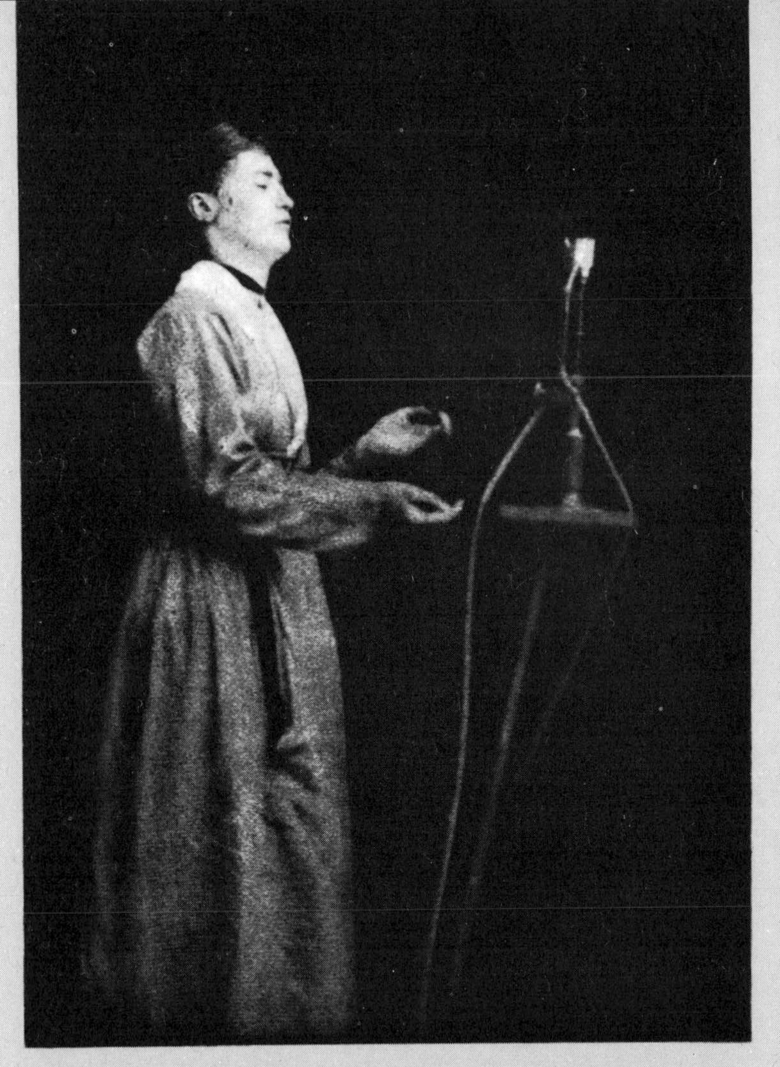

Planche XXII.

CATALEPSIE

PROVOQUÉE PAR UNE LUMIÈRE VIVE

A woman in a trance-state of catalepsy, induced by the action of light. Charcot used such demonstrations to confirm that hysteria and its symptoms were objective realities of the nervous system and of anatomy.

'body-in-itself' (Sartre), or 'the objective body' (Merleau-Ponty); Freud, on the other hand, believed that the pathogenesis of hysterical symptoms could only be understood through what the philosophers of this century have called 'interbody' (Ortega), 'the body-for-itself' (Sartre), or the 'phenomenal body' (Merleau-Ponty). In the first case, the disease never went beyond the phenomenological sphere of *what is in me*; in the second, the disease belonged more or less definitely and consciously to the phenomenological sphere of *what is mine*. From this it may be seen that this first subtle difference between Charcot and Freud, of January or February 1886, was the first historical occasion when the 'subjective' was introduced into medicine.

A few years later the disagreement between pupil and master became obvious and final, when Freud, now back in Vienna and collaborating with Breuer, began working on his own. In place of Charcot's concept of hysteria – visual, objective, conforming to type – Freud maintained a completely different attitude: auditory (in that it was not based on what the doctor saw when examining the patient's body, hysteria *ex visu,* but on what he heard when the patient spoke of his psyche, *hysteria ex auditu*), individualised (not conforming to type, but clinically and pathogenetically faithful to the maxim that 'every case is a case'), and subjective (attending to the patient's conscious and unconscious subjective state). Even from a sociological viewpoint, Charcot's hysteria differed from Freud's hysteria: the former was imitative, collective, hospital-minded and proletarian; the latter, original, individual, domestic and middle-class. Let the reader measure the sociol-

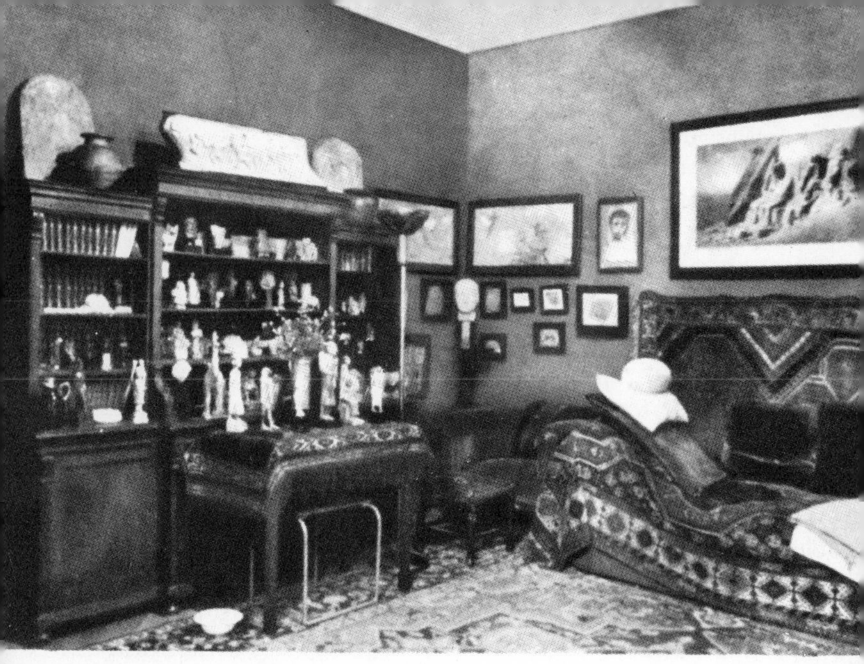

ogical difference between the surroundings in which Charcot and Freud worked – the former in a ward of the Salpêtrière full of hysterics in the *arc-de-cercle* position; the latter in his consulting-room in the Berggasse in Vienna – and he will have a clear picture of what was involved in the great sociological and psychological innovation of psychoanalysis.

As I said before, neurotic phenomena are the clinical signs of the 'rebellion of the subject' which preceded the introduction of the subjective element into medicine. We can now see that there was an apparent contradiction in the psychology of this 'rebellion'. Neurotics rebelled against the systematic and exclusively objective treatment they had been subjected to at the end of the nineteenth century, by being both obedient and disobedient. What else was the spectacular suggestibility of Charcot's hysterics except a sort of imitative and morbid

Freud's consulting-room in Vienna, where patients' illnesses were reported on as their personal property and as something unique to themselves.

obedience to the physician who was studying them? And how can we interpret their resistance to being cured, the contrast between the suggestible facility with which they 'produced' their illness and their obstinate resistance to the therapist's wishes, if not as unconscious disobedience to a form of therapy which ignored the subjective and personal nature of the diseased state under treatment? Obedient to the cause of their illness, disobedient to the unsuccessful attempts to cure it, the hysterics of the Salpêtrière collectively expressed the 'rebellion of the subject' against the purely objective attitude of nineteenth-century medicine.

Western medicine had from the first always been objective. And neurotic disorders – under whatever name – have certainly always existed, as is shown by the figures given in Sydenham's dissertation on hysteria. But it was only at the end of the nineteenth century that it became possible for such a distinguished clinician as Leube to say with all 'scientific' seriousness that the time a doctor gave to questioning his patient was completely wasted as far as a good diagnosis was concerned.[6] On the other hand, the historical and social causes previously referred to led to clinical pictures of neurosis becoming strikingly more frequent at the end of the nineteenth century and all through the twentieth. Unintentionally, and even unconsciously, it was Charcot more than anyone else who discovered this significant historical fact. To sum up: if the first sign of the introduction of the subjective element into medicine was the difference of opinion between Freud and Charcot concerning the localisation of hysterical paralyses, the social phenomenon presented by the Salpêtrière hospital was the first obvious manifestation of the rebellion of the subject to which this 'introduction' was the reply.

This is not the place to study Freud's later work and its influence on medical thought and practice during the twentieth century. I will merely mention early psychoanalytical studies of various organic diseases made by several of Freud's pupils (Groddeck, Ferenczi, Deutsch, 1918 to 1922); the study of 'organic neurosis' from the point of view of psychoanalysis and the psychology of the individual (in the book *Psychogenese und Psychotherapie körperlicher Symptome,* edited by Oswald Schwarz, Vienna 1925); Viktor von Weizsäcker's 'anthropological medicine'; the 'psychosomatic medicine' of the English-speaking world, and finally the gradual emergence of a new medical outlook, increasingly aware that without the systematic introduction of psychological and sociological methods into clinical practice, the sick cannot be understood and cared for scientifically.

For both clinical and social reasons the relation between doctor and patient was bound to become critical in the first half of the twentieth century; and this in fact is what has happened. Something no less important than the Hippocratic conversion of empirical and magic medicine into technical medicine has been occurring for the last few decades in medical science and the art of healing. Let us see what can be said today about this great innovation we are witnessing, and what is, what should be, and what can be the relation between doctor and patient in our day.

Part 2:
The doctor-patient relationship today

4 The basis of the relationship

The doctor-patient relationship of today is set in many different surroundings – the private consulting-room, the hospital ward, the public surgery-room of a socialised health service, the battlefield, and many other places. The patient may have been free to choose his doctor, or he may have been attended by the man assigned to him by the political, administrative or industrial organisation to which he belongs. Is there some common basis underlying these differences? I think there is, and that the lesson of ancient Greece has not been forgotten. Whether it is understood in a personal or social sense, whether it is regulated by a free contract between two individuals or by the rules of some welfare institution, if the link between doctor and patient is a correct one it will be based on philia between them – more specifically on 'medical philia' – to which the doctor contributes his desire to give technical help, and the patient his confidence in medicine and the doctor attending him. When this is not the case, something has gone wrong in the public or private practice of healing. Our problem consists in discovering exactly how 'medical philia' should be interpreted at the present time.

Medical care as a special form of help

Medical care of the sick is nowadays often carried out by a team; this is the necessary result of the complexity of modern medical techniques. But it naturally has to take the form of a series of medical 'events' – some diagnostic, others therapeutic – in each of which *one* member of the team, whether intern, surgeon, physiotherapist or psychiatrist, is brought into personal and direct contact with the patient. So that the team system has not led to the disappearance of a situation as old as medicine itself: technical care of the sick still definitely consists in one man helping another.

Of course there are many different forms of help. There is the mutual help given one another by comrades, or by friends and lovers. That between comrades, as we have seen, has as its aim some essentially external good of the two people involved; whereas friends and lovers seek communion by forming a single entity – a pair. To define these terms more exactly, we should say that the relation of mutual help is fulfilled in a *duo* in the former case, and in the latter a friendly or loving *diad*. There can also be unilateral help; in this case one person alone gives help and the other receives it. There seem to me three characteristic forms of help: advice, education and medical care.

In the *advisory relationship,* one man helps another to make an important *decision* in his life. It is the highest form of Heidegger's *Fürsorge,* or 'preventive care', in which one man, knowing the character of the other and guessing what he might become in the future, suggests a line of conduct but leaves him free either to take it or not to. It is for the man who receives the advice to decide whether to follow it. It is hardly necessary to say that, although formally distinct from friendship in the strict sense of the word, the advisory relation is closest amongst those I have named to the purely diadic relationships of friendship and love. It is perfectly possible for there to be a true philia in which neither of the two friends gives advice to the other, and it may also happen that the adviser is not the personal friend of the advised; but it is none the less certain that real friendship often has to be expressed in the form of advice, which is then the realisation of a diadic relationship.

In an *educational relationship*, the master helps his pupil to acquire the mental habit of learning and remembering. The highest standard of teaching requires some degree of philia: ever since the time of Socrates and Plato we have known that *erôs paidagôgikos,* psychologically and socially realised as *philia paidagôgikê,* is necessary to the art of education. But this 'educative philia' is not just interpersonal friendship, because while a friend respects his friend and gladly accepts him as he is without any diminution of good will, a teacher does not accept his pupil as he is, but as someone whose temporary deficiencies he is trying to remedy with his teaching. Therefore education is further from the diadic relationship than is the advisory relation.

Thirdly, we come to *medical care*. A doctor who helps a sick man is trying to help him attain a state of both mental and physical well-being – for this is what health consists of. And this requires detachment or objectivity, since in almost every illness, including those described as 'mental', the feelings the patient is experiencing and expressing to his doctor have an underlying physical cause. The doctor's friendship for his patient – medical philia – is thus even further than educative philia from pure interpersonal friendship.

Situated between the duo of comradeship and the diad of true friendship and love, these advisory, educational and medical relationships fulfil, each in their own way, a form of union between two people that I propose to call *quasi-diadic*. The co-operation between the members of a duo is wholly

Garibaldi, wounded at the battle of Aspromonte in August 1862, with his doctor Relaton.

based on their possessing a common purpose; between the members of a diad it is essentially based on carrying out together those psychic acts from which friendship and love are born and by which they express themselves. The result of this is that there may be dual relationships that are purely objective (like that between partners who are quite uninterested in each other's personal feelings), and diadic ones that are purely co-operative (like that between friends who do not care whether the other is tall or short, dark or fair). The dynamics of quasi-diadic relations differs from both these cases, because it necessitates a combination of objectivity and co-operation, though one or other may predominate. This is exactly what happens with a doctor, even at times when he is on mainly psychotherapeutic terms with his patient.

The doctor-patient relationship is thus a quasi-diadic and helpful co-operation, whose purpose is that the patient should achieve the psychosomatic situation we call health; of all helpful relations it is closest to what I have described as an objective one. But, as we shall soon see, its quasi-diadic character does not prevent its containing a social element.

We will go on now to investigate the inner structure of the medical relationship, leaving on one side for the moment those cases when it is confused in one way or another, and only considering those where the doctor acts with a sense of vocation and the patient with a real desire to get well, without any specially magical or superstitious attitude but with some confidence in the skill and moral honesty of the man who is attending him. In this sort of structure I distinguish four components: the proper aim of the relation, the proper form of

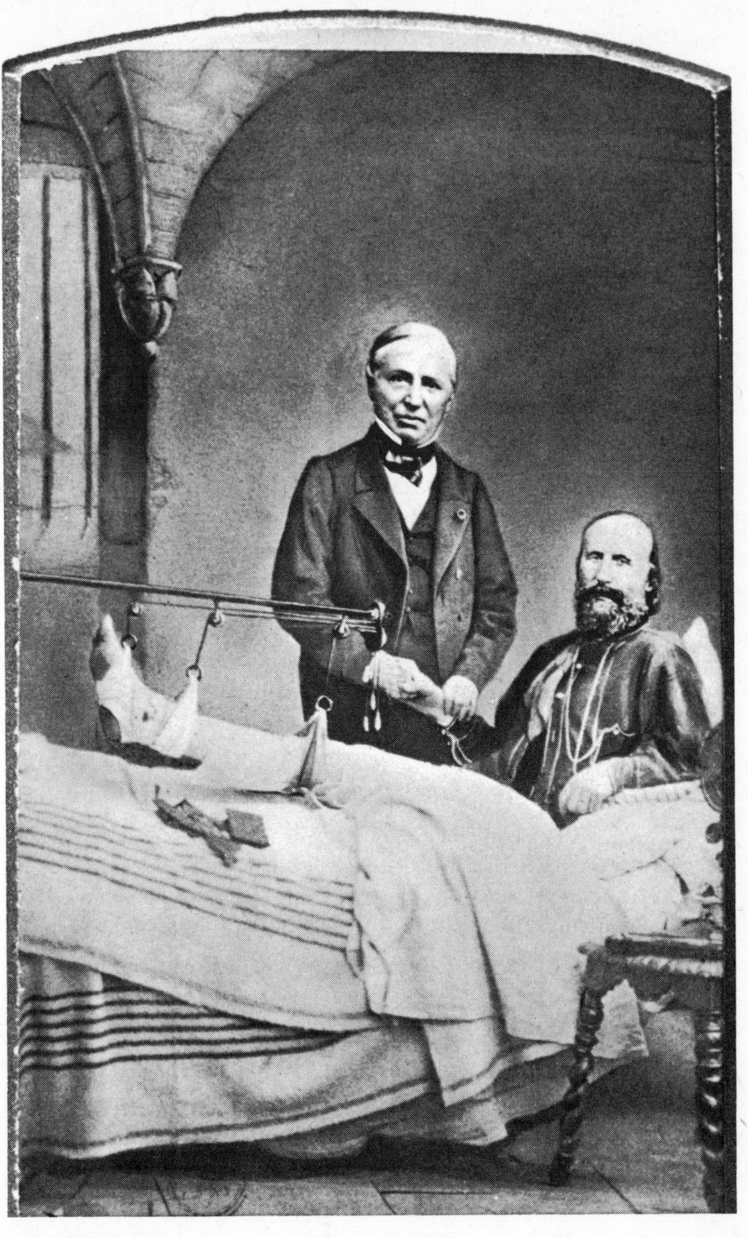

intercourse involved in it, the proper link on which this intercourse should depend, and lastly the proper form of communication between doctor and patient.

Components of the relationship

1 The proper aim of the medical relationship is the health of the patient; nothing could be more obvious than that. All the same, it is as well to emphasise the fact, because present-day medicine, intoxicated by its new and wonderfully effective techniques for controlling human nature, is sometimes led to believe that the doctor's ultimate aim may be man's moral goodness (to make men good) or the happiness of humanity (to make men happy), rather than the physical health of the invalid. The Utopian views expressed in Huxley's *Brave New World* have persisted and sprouted again with new strength in the West (since the Second World War in spite of Existentialism and *angst*). I have the greatest respect for science and technique but I am radically out of sympathy with this illusion. The doctor's proper task is not to make men good and happy but healthy. As a doctor, he cannot and he should not go beyond this. And since a healthy man is undoubtedly more likely to become good and happy than one who is ill or infirm, it would appear inherent in the human condition: first, that a man's goodness and happiness are not a necessary result of his health but depend on the use he makes of his liberty to build a life for himself, and on that mysterious factor controlling human life which the ancients called 'fate' and we call 'chance' or 'providence' according to our religious beliefs. And secondly, that the invariably imperfect conquest of these supreme

objectives should not be the doctor's responsibility but be undertaken by the individual himself, and by those whose job it is to organise society and formulate the ultimate aims of human life (politicians, teachers and priests). A healthy man can be good or wicked, sad or happy, according to the circumstances of his life, the use he makes of his freedom and his good or bad luck. I repeat: the proper aim of the relation between doctor and patient is for the patient to become healthy; or rather, as healthy as his individual constitution, his past history and the nature of the illness he is suffering from allow. This is the ultimate end to which the two subordinate branches of medical care known as 'diagnosis' and 'treatment' should always be directed.

2 The proper form of intercourse between doctor and patient, as I remarked before, consists in such a combination of objectivity and co-operation as is made necessary in each individual case by the diagnosis and treatment. In the process of diagnosis, objectivity is involved in finding a pulmonary cavity, or inflammation of the kidney, or in detecting an obsessional idea, and in treatment by means of gastrectomy, or the use of antibiotics. On the other hand co-operation is shown by psychologically reproducing in the mind of the doctor, insofar as that is possible, the meaning the patient's illness has for him. And of course, in his dealings with the patient, the doctor must supplement objectivity with co-operation and vice versa.

In the next chapter I shall show how this double task can be carried out. For the present I will confine myself to instancing

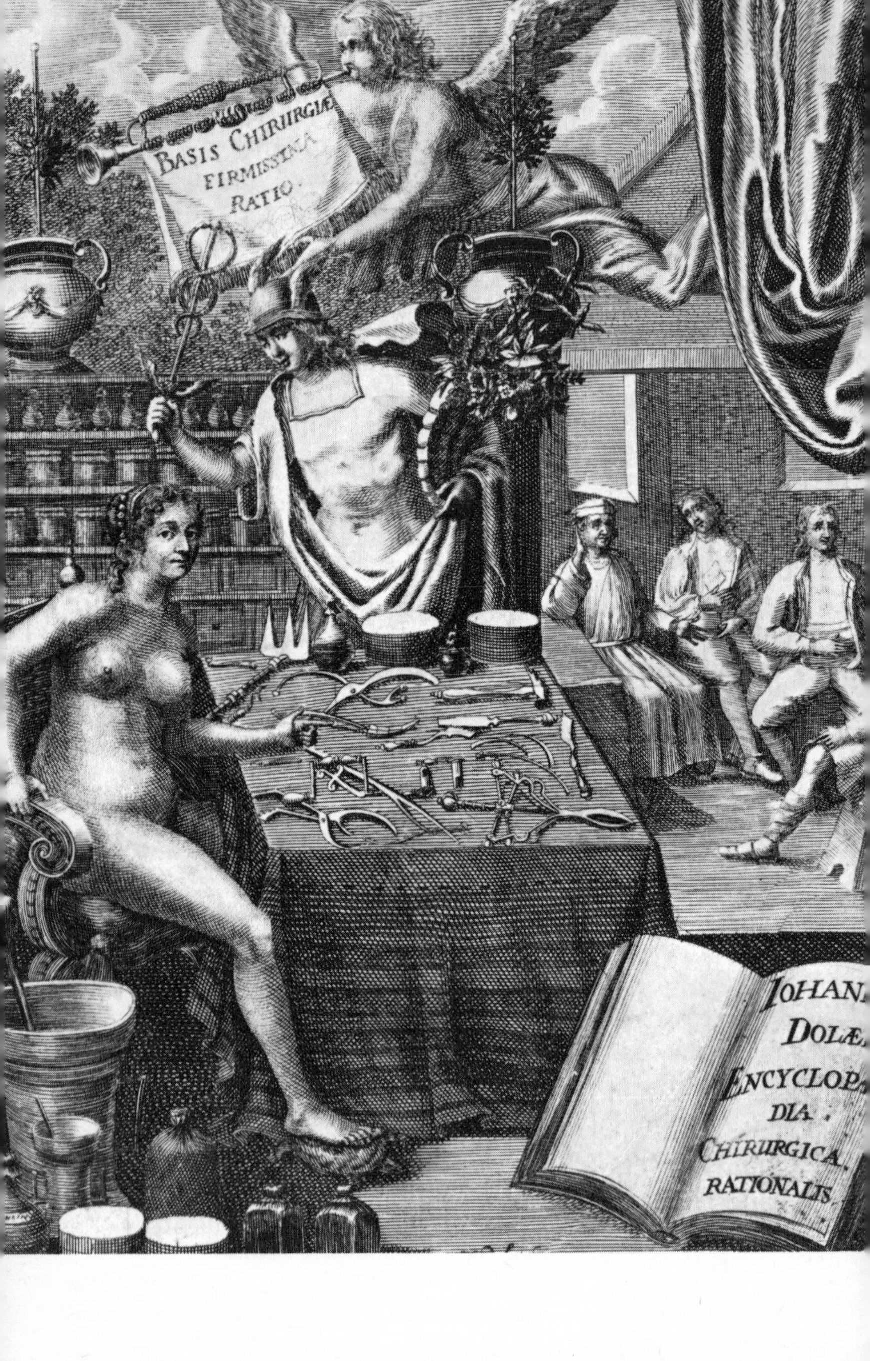
BASIS CHIRURGIÆ
FIRMISSIMA
RATIO.
IOHAN
DOLÆ
ENCYCLOPÆ
DIA.
CHIRURGICA
RATIONALIS

Seventeenth-century surgery found it necessary to defend itself against quackery. Appeals were often made to 'Reason', as in this frontispiece to Johann Dolaeus' surgical encyclopedia. Frankfurt, 1689. But today good surgery is marked as much by an understanding of an individual's response to its skills as by the objective knowledge that these take for granted.

an extreme case. Let us suppose that a surgeon is operating on the anaesthetised body of his patient, apparently a mere object, to be looked at, felt, incised and manipulated. In the course of this intervention, is it possible for a *good* surgeon to think and act towards the patient in a purely objective manner? Of course not. Leriche has more than once emphasised how important it is to imagine what the scar left on the patient's body by an operation will mean to him. In every case the incision must be made in such a way that the scar is as tolerable as possible, and this involves knowledge of the personality of the patient, his future existence and his reactions to the various eventualities of life – in fact it is necessary to co-operate imaginatively in the possible attitudes and responses of the *individual* whose body is being cut into by the scalpel.

The need for a doctor to be objective is obvious. But his co-operation – deliberate or otherwise – is no less necessary, although its actual importance varies according to whether the illness is acute, neurotic, or chronic.

In an *acute illness,* such as pneumonia, inflammation of the kidneys, etc., the possibility and medical value of co-operation between doctor and patient are minimal. With the exception of fear, the feelings produced by the illness – physical pain, vertigo, feverish weakness, etc. – are by their nature impossible to share. Toothache is felt by the sufferer and no one else, for which reason a purely objective diagnosis and treatment may be technically effective in such a case. But if diagnosis and treatment are to be perfect, surely it is necessary to enter into the part the illness is playing in the life of the patient? And does not such a knowledge, in the last resort imaginative and conjectural, depend on a purely co-operative attitude?

The case of *neurotic illness* is very different. For greater clarity, let us take a case of obsessional neurosis as an example. The doctor starts by listening to the patient's account of his troubles; as he listens he is *to some extent* understanding and mentally entering into the doubts and obsessions that the patient is living through in his own mind. But this co-operative or sympathetic diagnosis will not become a truly 'medical diagnosis' unless the clinician succeeds in a triple task of objectivation: namely, he must consider the patient's obsessional ideas as real 'mental entities', he must discover the psychological mechanism that has given rise to them, and – since the illness must surely have a physical aspect, though not always one that is apparent – he must attempt to discover the bodily change which was the immediate cause of the neurosis.

Between acute illness and neurosis, we find *chronic illness,* where the sufferer has to come to terms with his trouble and plan how his life is to be led. In such cases it is especially vital for the intercourse between doctor and patient to move from objectivity to co-operation, and from co-operation to objectivity, in other words the problem of medical care is at its most complicated, as we shall see later.

3 By the proper link on which the medical relation depends, I mean that which gives concrete reality to the objectivity and co-operation mentioned above. What is its special character? The answer cannot be a simple one, since the character of the link will depend on the intentions of the doctor and the attitude of the patient at their meetings. We shall soon see how many

possibilities there are. But disregarding their diversity for the present, we can say that, from the Hippocratics until the present day, it has repeatedly been declared that when medical care is what it should be, the link between doctor and patient is love. 'The deepest roots of medicine are in love,' to quote the lapidary phrase of Paracelsus. 'If our love is great, great will be the fruit it will obtain from medicine, but if it be lacking, the fruit will also be lacking. For it is love which causes us to learn the art, and no doctor can be created without it.'

I need not repeat here what I have written in earlier pages about the successive ways that 'medical philia' has been understood. I shall return to the theme later on; meanwhile I will only say that psychoanalysis has shown that the unique link technically described today as the 'transference' has much in common with the philia of the ancients. Here is Freud's first mention of it (in *Studies on Hysteria,* 1895):

> With other (patients) who have decided to put themselves in (the doctor's) hands and place their confidence in him – a step which in other such situations is only taken voluntarily and never at the doctor's request – ... it is almost inevitable that their personal relation to him will force itself, for a time at least, unduly into the foreground. It seems, indeed, as though an influence of this kind on the part of the doctor is a *sine qua non* to a solution of the problem.

Some years later, Freud gave the technical name of transference to this 'personal relation'.

4 The fourth component in the structure of the medical relation is the proper form of communication between those taking part in it: that is to say, the technical expedients used by

the doctor so that his objectivity and co-operation may take effect – observation, words and silence, manual and instrumental contact. To communicate with his patient the doctor must look at him, talk and listen, touch him with his hands and make use of a great number of different exploratory or therapeutic instruments. What each of these different means of communication represents in the connection between therapist and patient will be discussed later. We must however first examine the motives that control the meeting between the two.

The patient's and doctor's motives

The form taken by each particular case of the doctor-patient relationship mainly depends on the historical and social circumstances in which they meet; on the patient's personal attitude to his own illness, to medicine in general and his doctor; and on the doctor's personal attitude to the practice of his profession and to this particular patient. Let us concentrate for the present on the social aspect of the relationship, and consider what motives brought them together.

The patient's motives First, the patient. Here is a sick man. He may be in one of several situations: his own bed, a private consulting-room, a public surgery. Whatever the circumstances, can we classify his motives for meeting the doctor? Three separate questions must be answered:

1 *What was the sick man's aim when he sought medical aid?* This question also must be divided into three, according to the

The stethoscope, a technical expedient in medical communication. Dr Laennec (1781–1826), its inventor, examines a patient at the Hospital Becker, Paris. After a fresco by Theobald Chartran in the Sorbonne.

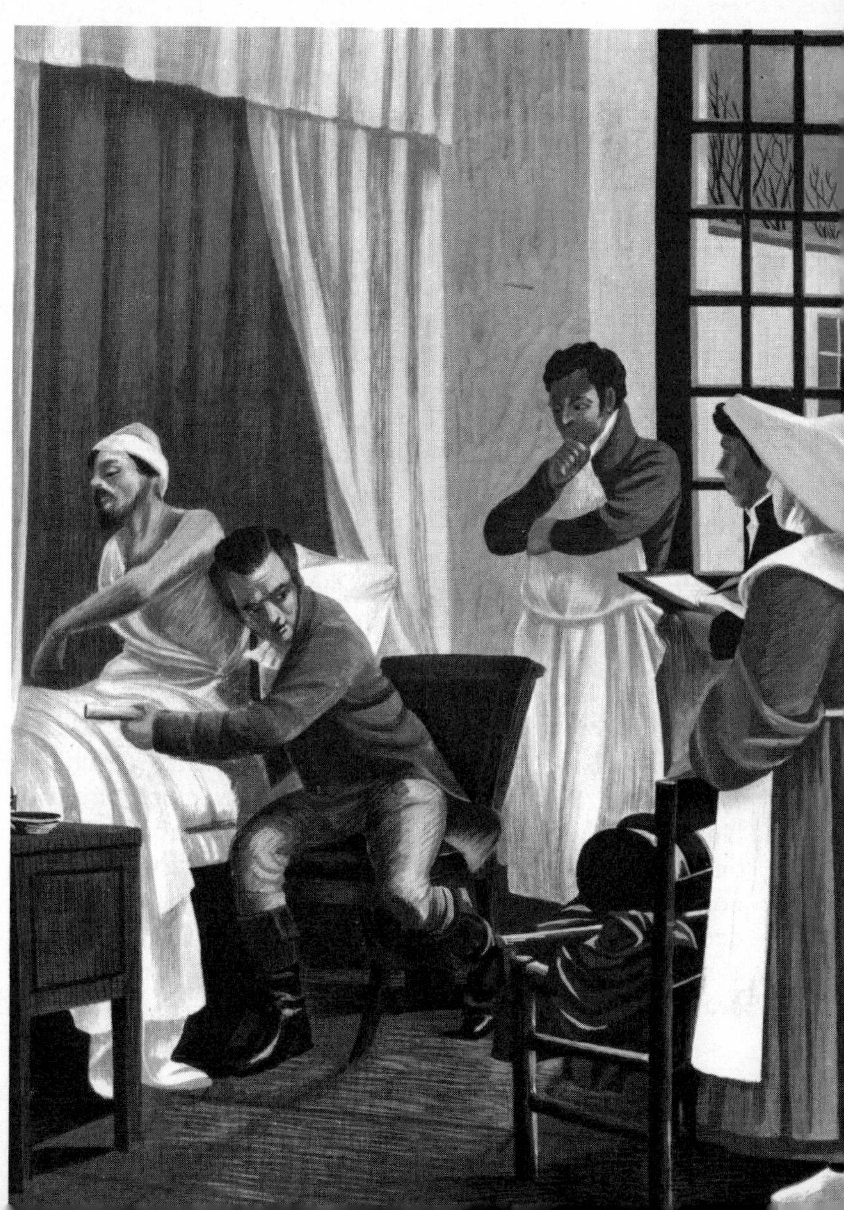

class of motives involved: those affecting the invalid himself, his social surroundings and the choice of doctor.

In general, the sick man has consulted the doctor because he wants to get well; the desire for health is the most frequent of all the motives affecting the invalid himself. One must not forget, however, that there are degrees and ways of desiring health. Some patients long passionately to be well again, and their longing exists at both a conscious and an unconscious level. There are others whose desire for health is lukewarm, either out of habitual or temporary lack of vitality or some other special reason. Finally, there are some in whom a discrepancy can be observed between their conscious and unconscious attitudes; sometimes beneath apparent indifference to their own health there exists a strong desire to get well and to live, at other times what at first sight looks like a conspicuous desire for health really conceals a more or less acute *taedium vitae* in the deeper regions of the self.

But desire to regain lost health is not always the principal motive that sends the invalid to his doctor. There are cases in which the dominant motive is desire for a diagnosis, an urgent need to 'know what is the matter'. The strength of modern man's impulse to 'know where he stands' usually strengthens this motive, even when the patient is very much afraid of illness. An educated man of today nearly always insists on being given a detailed diagnosis, and it is in search of this – not only in search of health – that he goes to consult his doctor. So, sometimes, does a peasant. Dr Garcia-Sabell's medico-anthropological observations on the Galician peasantry are relevant here.[7]

Sometimes another motive dominates the sick man's mind: a more or less conscious intention of taking refuge in illness, and therefore refuge in the doctor. It is hardly necessary to mention how intensely this motive is seen in the compensation neurosis or in battle neurosis, but there is no need to have recourse to such extreme examples in order to discover how real it is or how frequently it occurs even in apparently well-balanced individuals.

There remain those cases when the man who consults his doctor does not feel ill. The two most important instances of this seem to be: when he goes for a routine examination or check-up, to use the wide-spread modern term, in order to confirm his healthy state or discover some as yet undiagnosed diseased condition; and secondly, simulation, or an attempt to deceive the doctor with fictitious symptoms. A careful and sensitive practitioner will realise the great importance of the problem of simulation. Where does simulation begin and end? Is an individual who deliberately and skilfully imitates sciatica or amblyopia for the doctor's benefit merely a malingerer? To answer this last question in the affirmative is in my opinion over-simple.

Next we come to motives concerning the patient's social environment. Even when the decision to 'go and see the doctor' or 'call in the doctor' seems to be an autonomous and personal one, it always contains a hidden reference to other people. The patient may be aware of it or not, but there are always 'others' present in his mind – his wife, children, parents and so on – when he decides to seek medical aid, and a good clinician is always interested in the secret world of his patient's intentions.

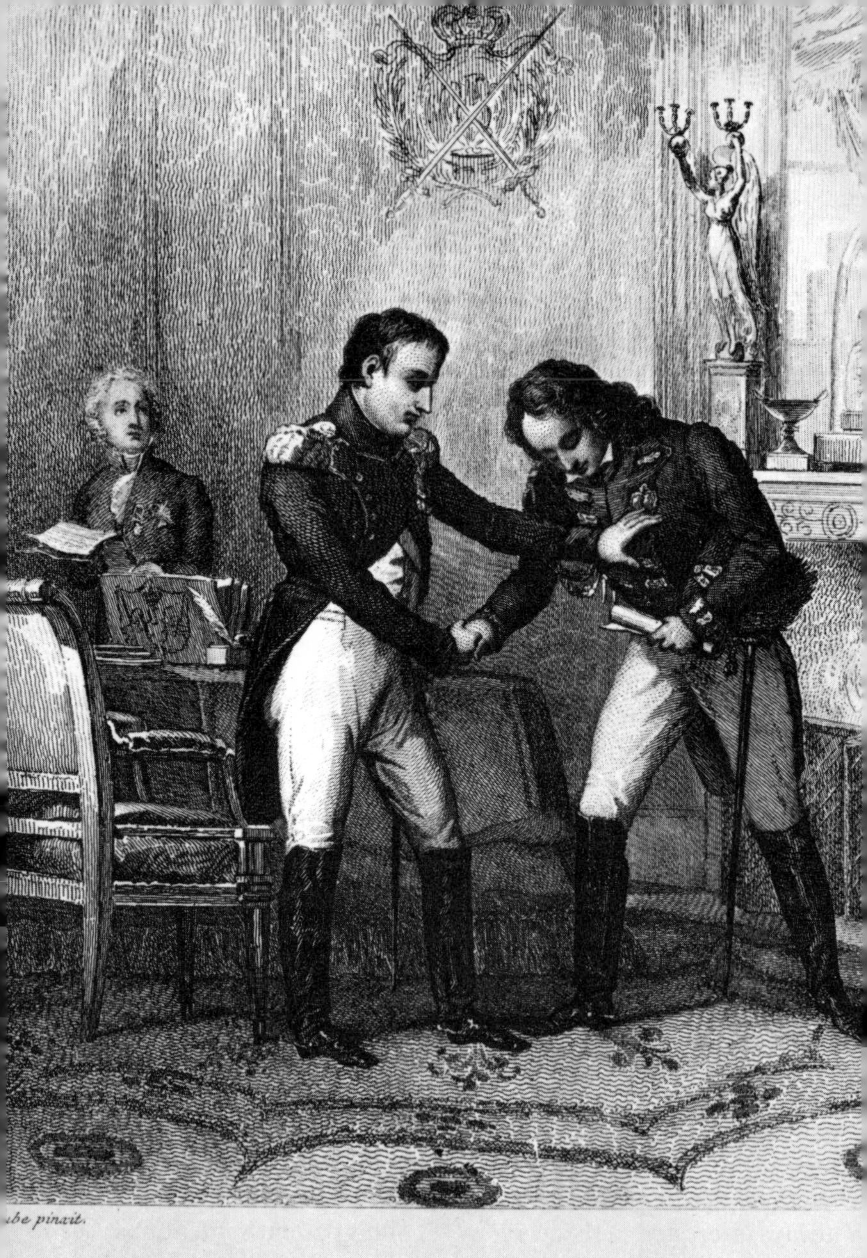

…abe pinxit.

L'Empereur dit à Larrey: "Je serais bien heureux de n'être entouré que par des hommes tels que vous.

Napoleon and Baron Larry, his physician.
'I would be very happy to have
only such men as you around me.'
After a painting by Steuben.

The impulse may have been set going by his 'next of kin' – the members of his own family who surround the invalid and are in direct contact with him – or by those numerous impersonal and collective 'others' who make up society. The invalid may then be impelled towards the doctor by the influence of the social group to which he belongs. If a society has a flourishing interest in hygiene, its citizens will have to submit to various exploratory or preventive measures. If it is dominated by economic considerations, its citizens will have certain medical obligations as workers. A soldier's career imposes other conditions. Sometimes it is the responsibility attached to the patient's important position in society. We have an example in Ernst von Bergmann's memoirs, which describe the medical treatment given to the Emperor Frederick III of Germany soon after his coronation for the cancer of the larynx which caused his death. The case would have been treated quite differently if he had been an ordinary person. From the outset it was clear that he had a cancer, but for reasons of state it could not be diagnosed openly.

Lastly, there are motives concerning the choice of doctor. In search of health, a diagnosis, or a refuge for his defencelessness, the patient has decided either of his own accord or for other reasons, to 'go and see a doctor' or 'call in a doctor'. Whom will he go to, whom will he call in? There are four typical solutions:

(a) He chooses *a certain doctor*, because of his public reputation. This should in principle give the best chance of a medically favourable meeting.

(b) The patient goes to *the doctor*. A previous commitment, engaged upon freely or otherwise – a contractual agreement, membership of some health organisation, or the fact of living in a small village – may direct the patient's need towards a certain doctor. He has not chosen the man who is to look after him, but he knows him before calling on his services.

(c) The patient accepts *the doctor he is offered* although he does not know him; he is provided by the health organisation he is obliged to belong to as a worker, civil servant or soldier. In such cases the organisation, whatever it may be, stands between doctor and patient, and according as its reputation is good or bad it will be favourable or disturbing to the therapeutic relation.

(d) The patient has recourse to *any doctor* who happens to be available in his moment of need. This is certainly not the most propitious start for medical treatment, but some of the circumstances involved – the patient's urgent need, lack of prejudice in his relation with the doctor, who becomes merely a personification of 'medicine' or 'science', are not altogether unfavourable to the success of the treatment – assuming of course that the physician in question is technically adequate.

2 *How did the patient begin to feel ill?* The 'how' of this question naturally refers to the onset of the 'feeling of illness', a subject given little importance by traditional pathology and clinical medicine, but receiving increasing attention from modern doctors. I will briefly examine the structure and genesis of this feeling.

In the actual structure of the feeling of being ill one must distinguish the conscious experience from physiological mechanisms. The generic feeling of being ill – that which generically unites all possible individual sensations of illness – pain, vertigo, feverish weakness, inability to move, obsessional ideas, anxiety, amnesia, etc. – is not a simple experience. With one or the other element preponderating, there appear to me as many as seven quite distinct experiences concerned: disability, discomfort, awareness of danger, absorption in bodily sensations, loneliness, the sense of being different and the feeling of refuge. By *disability* I here mean partial or total inability to carry out some of the functions necessary to normal human life. In every illness there is in fact an element of 'I can't'. *Discomfort* is the generic and direct affliction of being ill, including physical pain in the strict sense, anxiety, depression, etc. Illness also brings with it an awareness of *danger;* the sense of being at death's door of Heidegger's ontological analyses is a conscious or subconscious psychological experience, according to circumstances, and resulting from illness. By *absorption in bodily sensations* I mean that the ailing body imperiously attracts all the individual's attention, including his mental life. This is the cause of the peculiar *loneliness* of the invalid. Illness mentally isolates him. The sense of being *different* is the psychological correlative of the 'abnormality' of objective pathology: the invalid feels 'different' from the healthy people surrounding him. Finally, the state of being ill is felt as a *refuge*: the patient does not think of his suffering only in terms of disability, affliction, threat and isolation; it is in some way useful to him.

Disability, discomfort, sense of danger, absorption in the body, solitude, sense of being different, refuge; these are the

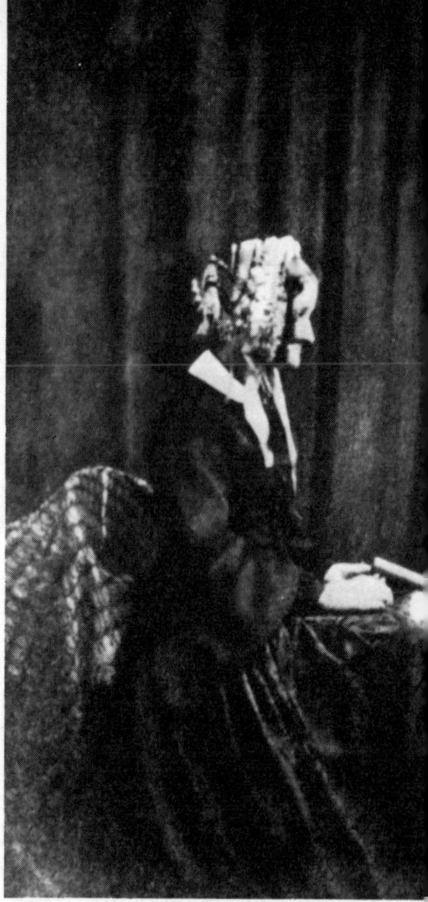

This photograph ('Fading Away') apparently shows a girl dying of an incurable disease, and well illustrates many elements and sensations in being ill. For 1858, it was a shocking idealisation of a tragic subject. In fact the photograph was a composite, from five different negatives, and the patient a fine healthy girl made up to seem on the point of death.

integral states of mind making up the generic feeling of illness. They are present in every sick person, although some may be more apparent than others. Added to them and colouring them are those symptoms arising from the special disease he suffers from (pneumonia, gastric ulcer, etc.), and those depending on his own personality and constitution – sex, age, and so on. All these sensations must be derived from the activity of those organs that enable us to be aware of our own bodies, external

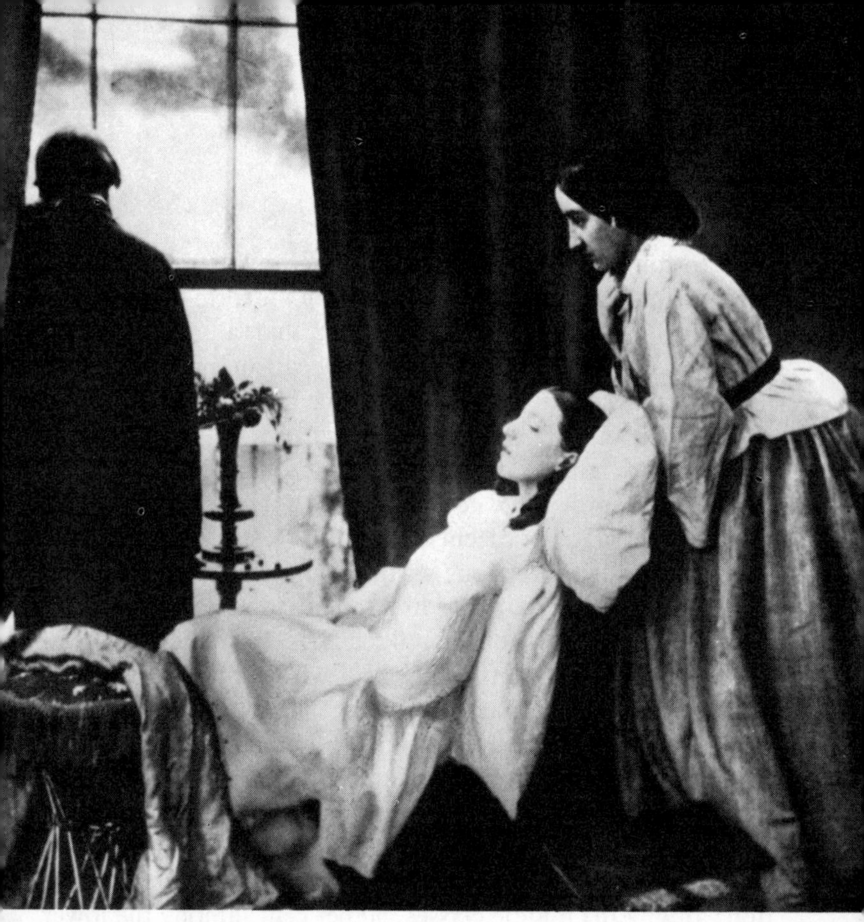

and internal receptors, the autonomic nervous system, the brain itself, reticular system, hypothalamus, mesencephalon and cortex. These are the chief components of the *neurophysiological mechanism* involved in a sense of being ill.

In psychological terms, the *genesis* of the feeling of illness is the transition from a sense of 'well-being' belonging to health – consisting in having no painful awareness of one's body – to the 'uneasiness' of the state of illness. It will not be out of place to comment here on the importance of historico-cultural situation and economico-social status in the form taken by the feeling of illness. How can the fact that a man's mental attitude is either predominantly magical, or predominently rational and scientific, fail to influence his manner of feeling ill? The Tongas of Africa believe that intestinal worms are necessary to human digestion; in certain South American tribes skin disorder, *mal de los pintos,* is not considered to be a disease at all (Ackerknecht); nor, in the strict sense of the word, were such infections as trachoma by Greek peasants until a few years ago, according to Lawson's medico-sociological researches. As for the influence of economic and social status on the genesis of feeling ill, I will merely mention the convincing findings made by Koos. This writer studied the relation between social class and those symptoms that are taken as indicating disease: loss of appetite, repeated attacks of lumbar pain, chronic cough, persistent pain in the muscles and joints, excessive menorrhagia, etc. Among the upper classes, 57 per cent thought loss of appetite a morbid condition; among the middle classes, 50 per cent; among the lower classes, 20 per cent. Even more significant are the figures relating to chronic cough (77 per cent in the upper classes, 23 per cent in the lower classes) and pains in joints and muscles (80 per cent and 19 per cent) and other subjective and objective symptoms. The reader will be reminded of the incisive passages in Plato attacking those luxury-loving citizens who sent for the doctor for the slightest discomfort.

3 *How did the patient respond to feeling ill?* Before he decided

A society's culture influences its members' attitude to illness, even to the way such illness is felt. An Eskimo shaman, in a trance, draws the sickness from his patient's head with a stave.

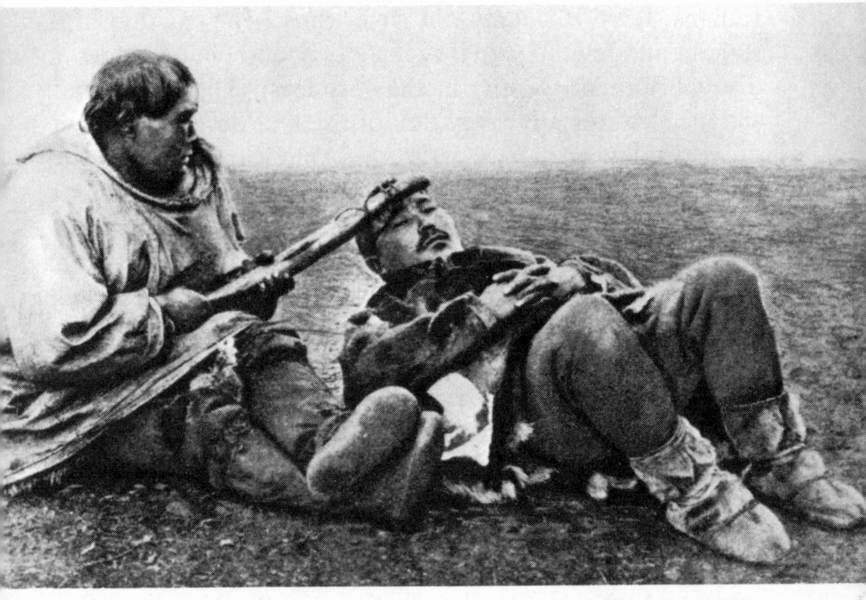

whether to consult the doctor or not, what passed through his mind about his feeling of illness? I think three aspects of the patient's response should be distinguished, the affective, the interpretative and the operative. In its *affective aspect* his response to his feeling of illness may adopt many different forms: rebellion against it, resigned acceptance, depression, apathy, anxiety, despair, concealed pleasure, infantilism, and many others. Let us take pain for example. How does the sufferer respond to it? M. Zborowski has studied the ways in which members of different groups behave when in pain:

Italians, Jews, Irish and 'old Americans'. The reaction of the Italians and Jews to pain is exaggerated; complaining does not disqualify them socially in the very least. The Irish usually suffer more stoically; they do not think it 'decent' to make a great display of pain. Lastly, the Americans try to be 'objective' about pain. All this, as Zborowski himself stresses, has a decisive influence on the relation between the patient and the doctor attending him. The patient's response also has an *interpretative aspect*: he is to some extent interpreting his feeling of illness. In the course of history, man has interpreted illness in four typical ways: as punishment, chance, a challenge or a test. At times men have believed (for instance, in Assyria and Babylonia, Ancient Greece, Israel) that illness expiated some crime they had committed; at others that it was the result of some unfortunate and incomprehensible fatality (illness as misfortune or *a-tychia,* as in the *Encomium of Helen* by Gorgias, or *La Peste* by Camus), or a challenge to man's powers of invention and skill (this was the proper interpretation of scientific medicine according to the Hippocratics), or that it was a test in which the patient could acquire personal merit or the reverse (the Christian attitude). Besides its affective and interpretative aspects, the response to the feeling of being ill has an *operative aspect*. The patient in fact communicates his state to other people or keeps silent about it, decides to stay in bed or remain up and about, engages in some magical, religious or scientific practice, consults or does not consult his doctor, etc. Let us consider the state of a sick man in this predicament. He feels ill. He responds affectively and interpretatively. Afterwards he decides to go to the doctor, more exactly to some special doctor, *the* doctor, or *a* doctor. What will be his preliminary attitude to the man who is to treat him technically? All the motives we have studied in the preceding pages will combine to stimulate his response.

The doctor's motives We must now briefly examine the doctor's motives when he meets the man who is to be his patient. Whatever the situation in which the meeting takes place – the invalid's house, the hospital, a public or private consulting-room, a battlefield, etc. – can the doctor's various motives be systematically classified? As in the previous case I will divide the theme into three questions.

1 *How does the doctor become the special sort of doctor he is?* Three combined elements can be distinguished in the formation of an individual – vocation, training and practice. His vocation as a doctor is the product of a greater or less inclination to help those in need, and therefore the sick, combined with what might be called a sporting instinct for overcoming natural difficulties by scientific and technical means. Only someone in whom these two vocational aspects are present can be a really good doctor. Of course some doctors have a very strong vocation and others a defective one. The doctor's technical training, which may have been good or bad, gives shape and efficacy to this vocational disposition. And both these, vocation and training, function operatively and socially in his practice – that is to say in his private and social method of understanding and practising medicine. In chapter 3 I described the four cardinal modes of the medical

The vital sympathy of a good doctor.
In Ruanda Urundi, Dr Vyncke works with
African patients in a psychiatric ward.

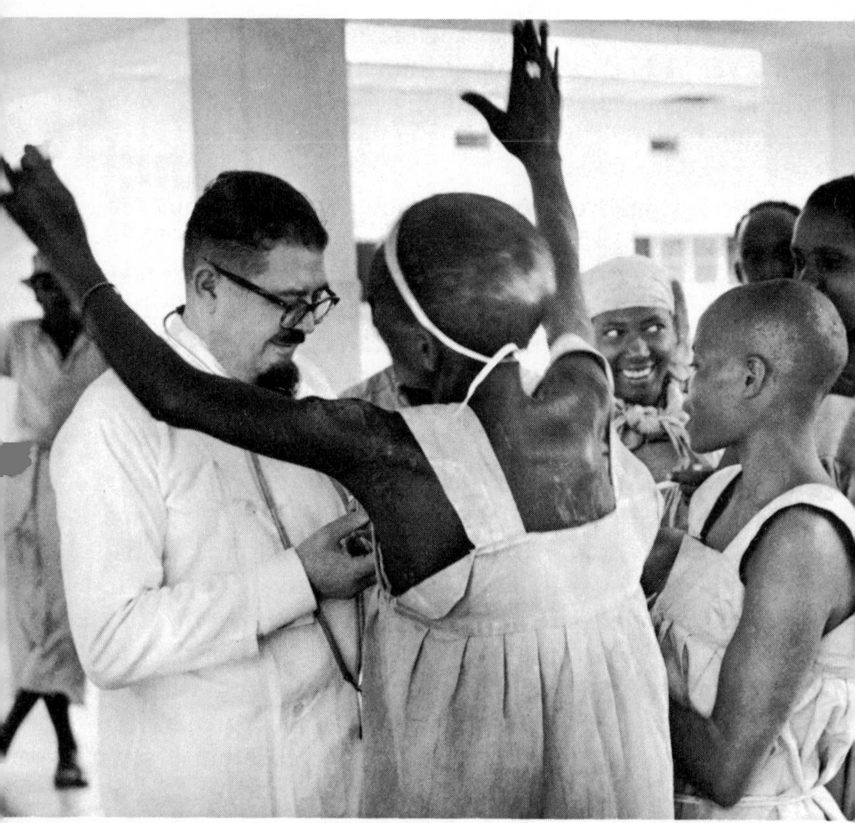

profession corresponding to the practitioner's chief motives: scientific knowledge, financial reward, the desire to carry out the most noble of all professional duties, and the impulse to give technical help to those in need of it.

2 *What sort of individual is the doctor?* Would an ideal doctor be a special sort of man? In other words, is there a 'medical personality'? In principle, given a certain talent and a minimal vocation, any man can be a doctor. But this is not to deny that certain temperamental, intellectual and moral qualities are necessary for a 'good doctor'. One of these is vital sympathy, that warm and welcoming glow that puts almost everyone at his ease. It can be said of men who are well-endowed with this quality that they are 'natural doctors', to twist Tertullian's well-known expression. Among intellectual qualities, is a capacity for comparative observation, and for entering into the mental state of other people imaginatively; among moral qualities, a constantly benevolent disposition, and that readiness to invent unwritten duties so often praised by Marañon. Much can be achieved by anyone who sincerely and steadfastly wishes to acquire these essential characteristics for a good doctor. *Quod natura non dat, Salmantica non praestat*; the old proverb rightly stresses that what nature herself does not provide will hardly be acquired at the university. But it is also true that: *Quod natura non dat, bona voluntas praestat.* The truth of this is plain to anyone with his eyes open.

3 *What is the doctor's attitude to the patient he is going to help?* If the doctor already knows the patient, his attitude will

be based on experience. 'So Smith's got his indigestion again', he may sometimes say to himself. But he often knows nothing about the patient he is going to treat. Will he be a 'good patient'? Or is he going to be a 'nuisance'? The situation, his idea of himself, and the occasion will condition the doctor's attitude. The situation: whether he practises his profession in convenient or inconvenient surroundings. His idea of himself: whether he is confident in his own technical adequacy or not. The occasion: the special moment in his life when this medical encounter takes place. How often are the shortcomings of the doctor-patient relationship due to the fact that the doctor is just about to go on holiday, for example?

Doctor and patient, each influenced by his own motives, are about to meet. The characters have taken their places on the stage and the curtain is going up. What comedy or drama will result from such a meeting? How will the basis of this mutual relationship – 'medical philia' in the most favourable circumstances – express itself in examination, diagnosis, and treatment? Let us see.

5 The structure of the relationship

We shall consider in turn communication between doctor and patient, and the affective, cognitive, operative, ethical and social aspects of the medical relationship.

Communication between doctor and patient

As soon as doctor and patient meet, they begin to communicate: they look at each other, talk and listen; and through technical resources of examination – inspection, history-taking, manual and instrumental examination – the clinician begins to establish his diagnosis and a scientific basis for treatment.

1 Before anything else happens, doctor and patient look at each other. What is taking place between them? According to Sartre, a look exchanged between two men is *essentially* an attempt at reciprocal objectivation, a conflict between two freedoms in which each tries to turn the other into a mere 'object'. 'Every glance is an act of aggression' wrote Ernst Jünger. But this is not always true. The purpose of a person looking at another need not be purely objective, and the looks exchanged between doctor and patient exemplify this fact.

When the patient trusts his doctor, he usually approaches him with a pleading expression. He does not see him as an object occupying space and time, but as a source of help, and not susceptible to calculation. If the relation between them is an ideal one, the patient does not think of the doctor in terms of planning, but of hope. However, at times the expression in the patient's eyes may also be demanding, objective, or even defiant.

Usually more complex than the patient's, the doctor's gaze – or that of the good doctor – normally expresses three main purposes: first, an enveloping purpose, by which it provides a haven of refuge for the patient's state of need. Just as a gaze can be a prison it can also be a haven, and so it should be in the doctor's case. Secondly, an inquisitive purpose, directed to the patient's body as a whole and in detail, and using the expressive signs made by it to read his inner feelings, the invisible world of his thoughts and his conscious and unconscious intentions. Thirdly, an objective purpose. When the doctor finds what he is looking for, or something he was not looking for, his gaze must treat the discovery 'objectively', although – for this to be truly 'medical' – he must do so within the broad context of the purpose I have called 'enveloping'. The clinician should never look at his patient as an entomologist looks at an insect. In short, by looking at the patient, the doctor *perceives* some part of his objective reality, and also *contributes* something to it.

It does not seem to me irrelevant to postulate the need for clinical 'optitechnique' of this sort. A doctor is taught how to observe, how to ausculate and test reflexes. It is just as important for him to learn how to look at the patient, so that he is not only subjecting him to the sort of inspection described in text books of symptomatology, but is also taking human and personal factors into account.

2 Besides looking at each other, doctor and patient talk together. It must be remembered that the conversation between them is always diagnostic and therapeutic at the same

time, in spite of the fact that the history-taking, which is predominantly diagnostic, is for technical reasons traditionally kept separate from verbal psychotherapy (conversation that is predominantly therapeutic in purpose). For the moment I propose to consider the first.

The *form* of taking a history (a 'dialogue') must be distinguished from the *content* (what is being said to each other by patient and doctor).

As to form, the patient's share of the interview is made up of audible paraverbal expressions, verbal expressions in the strict sense (words) and silences.

I call audible paraverbal expressions all those phonetic elements of the conversation that fall short of being words: sighs, deep breathing, exclamations – repressed or otherwise – drawn-out consonants, nasal pronunciation of certain syllables, interruptions and so forth. With the help of an expert in linguistics, C. F. Kockett, two psychiatrists, R. E. Pittenger and J. Danehy, have shown the great importance of such paraverbal phonemes during a clinical interview, especially during the first few minutes.[8]

However, this in no way diminishes the overruling importance of verbal expression proper. What function does the mere utterance of words, independently of what they say, perform in the medical relation? In an already classic description, the psychologist Karl Bühler distinguished three principal functions of words: the 'vocative' or 'calling of attention', the 'expressive' or 'informative', and the 'nominative' or 'representational'. Anyone who talks to someone else is calling on his attention, informing him of something and naming that thing. Nothing could be more obvious and illuminating. But to my mind this excellent classification of Bühler's should be completed in two ways. Above all, by adding another to these three functions of language – the 'persuasive'. Anyone talking to another person, merely by speaking, subjugates and persuades him (or anti-persuades, if the expression is not too displeasing and awkward). Secondly, Bühler's scheme is incomplete because it only takes account of the action as completed by the hearer and not its passive reverse function – what is liberated in the speaker's mind by speech.

The correlative of the vocative function is 'sodality' or company: calling on another person's attention makes us begin to live in his company. The correlative of the 'informative' function is the 'liberating' or 'cathartic' function: communicating something to another person brings a feeling of relief and tranquillity. The inner correlative of the nominative function is illumination: naming what is in our consciousness organises and lights up the mind to some extent. And the seductive or persuasive function of language is matched with a self-assertive one in the mind of the speaker; by speaking to someone else he is asserting himself. A sick person is no exception to this general rule. Thus, when he talks to the doctor, merely by the act of speaking he is appealing to him, informing him of something, naming that thing more or less exactly, and persuading or dissuading him of something; and at the same time he is receiving companionship, relieving his feelings, illuminating his own mind, and in a sense asserting himself. No consultation can be effective unless the doctor keeps this state of things in mind.

A clinical dialogue does not consist only of verbal and paraverbal phonemes; there are also silences on the part of both patient and doctor. It would be difficult to exaggerate the importance of silence in human life, and as a consequence in the relation between patient and doctor. Sometimes the patient is silent for negative reasons: because he does not know how, or is unable or unwilling to say something which is in his mind at the moment. But at other times his reasons are genuinely positive. There may be significant silences on the patient's part, when he stops speaking in order to give expression wordlessly to events and realities that are painful to him to expose openly; or trans-significant silences, when the experience of being ill forces him to confront the ultimate facts of his own life, and therefore his own death. A patient's silence when in the company of his doctor can be a serious or even momentous subject.

The doctor's participation in the dialogue is also formally speaking made up of paraverbal sounds, words and silences. The doctor should limit his use of involuntary paraverbal expressions as much as possible, make those that are voluntary as slight as possible, whether vocal or gestural, and choose those (such as inflections and cadences of voice, pauses, etc.) which help to show his desire to offer a 'haven of refuge' to the patient's need. He will, above all, fulfil the four active functions of language mentioned above (vocative, informative, nominative and persuasive) and he will control his conversation with the patient by using them to question, explain and orient gently and discreetly. But the doctor must also 'be able to hold his tongue'. By saying nothing, but listening to the patient attentively and kindly, the doctor is both getting to know him and curing him, because only when they are heard in silence do words fully reveal their meaning, and – above all – because nothing is more soothing than that haven of silence offered by one who says nothing to the speaker. A good clinician knows how to avoid useless digressions on the patient's part, and never forgets this double and subtle function of good listening.

Hitherto we have studied anamnesis from the formal point of view, insofar as it is a dialogue; now we shall go on to consider it from the point of view of the *content* of that dialogue. What do doctor and patient say to each other in the course of this history-taking? What significance have their remarks to the relationship established between them?

Let us look first at what the patient says in words and silence. Unless he wastes time digressing, he is speaking of himself as an invalid, and of everything in his life that has a bearing on his sufferings. But he can and does in fact adopt two different and complementary ways of talking: one testifying and the other interpreting. In the first he testifies to himself and his life; in the second he interprets his illness.

When what he says takes the form of testimony, the patient is contemplating his own condition objectively, and talking about it almost exactly – insofar as that is possible – as if he were speaking of someone else. This is what is happening when someone says to his doctor 'My ankles are swollen', or 'I had scarlet fever when I was a child'. This testimony can be of three different sorts. The patient can be a witness to his own external surroundings (as when he says to the doctor, to explain how a fracture has been caused, 'A lorry ran into me'), or to his own body (contemplating it from without, 'I developed a red rash'; or from within, 'I have a stomach-ache'), or to his inner feelings (when he tells the doctor about his depression, fears, hopes, or desperation).

Particularly since Freud's day, clinical anamnesis has become an interpretative communication. The patient does not only tell the doctor what he sees and feels (or saw and felt) in himself and his surroundings; he also tells him what this means to him. For example, read what Frau Emmy von N. said to Freud about the meaning of her remarks 'Be quiet! Don't talk to me! Don't touch me!' Since the diagnosis of a neurosis can only be interpretative, the doctor must start by considering the patient's interpretations of his own illness, even if they appear incorrect or capricious. And what illness, even the most purely somatic, does not include some more or less neurotic component in its clinical picture? The patient's interpretation may be 'constructive' or 'symbolical'. In the former, he explains to the doctor his personal view of the significance of his sufferings. In the latter, he consciously or unconsciously condenses into an expressive symbol his personal attitude to his illness or to one of his symptoms. Freud, Jung and Adler have taught us to recognise and evaluate the symbolical expressions of the sick.

If we bear in mind that the object of the patient's communications, whether as testimony or interpretation, may be present reality (auto-inspection) or past reality (autoretrospection). I think we can tabulate this communicative activity as follows:

Freud working on his *Outlines of Psychoanalysis* in 1938. History-taking has become more important since Freud realised that a patient's own testimony adds (constructively or symbolically) to the objective view taken by the doctor. Such testimony can help even with purely physical symptoms.

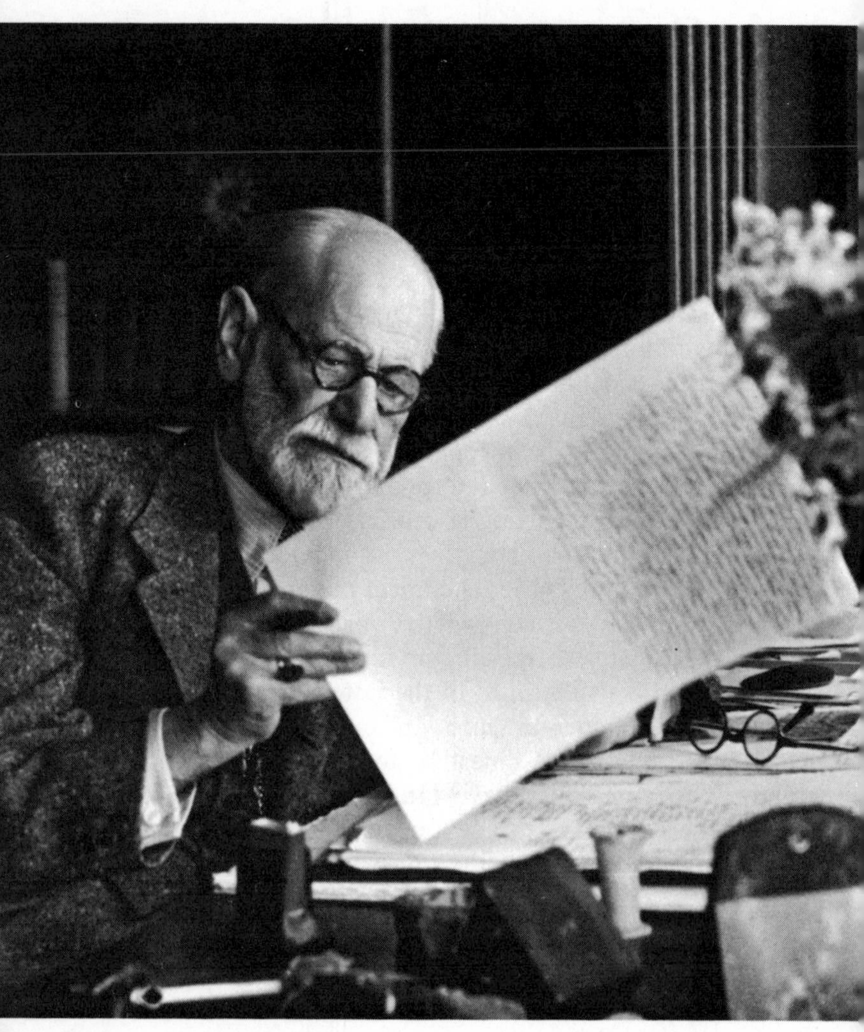

First, the patient talks to the doctor as

a witness	of his surroundings of his own body of his inner state	introspectively retrospectively
		through paraverbal expression through words through silence

Secondly, the patient talks to the doctor as

an interpreter	of his surroundings of his own body of his inner state	introspectively retrospectively
		through constructive interpretation through symbolical interpretation

We must now consider the content of what the doctor expresses in words and in silence. The patient talks about his illness and himself. The doctor, on the other hand, must not talk about himself, but about the patient and his illness. How? By applying the following methods to the particular case:

(a) *Interrogation.* The doctor questions the patient about everything in his external and internal life that concerns the genesis, configuration and significance of his illness.

(b) *Stimulation.* The doctor stimulates the patient to continue his account and amplify it with further facts.

(c) *Orientation.* The patient embarks on useless digressions.

(d) *Suggestion.* Without necessarily taking the form of verbal psychotherapy, the doctor's remarks will aim at encouraging the patient all the time. Nor will he forget the Hippocratic teaching that the patient will think him the worst doctor in the world 'if he does not promise to cure what is curable and to cure what is incurable' (*De morbis,* I. 6; L. VI, 150). 'Do not promise health', only 'fidelity and diligence', as Arnaldus de Vilanova said. Do not say 'of course' too often, but rather 'I will do my best', is the advice given by R. H. Blum in our own time.

(e) *Instructions.* These must always be given in a tone of invitation: 'Breathe deeply', 'Say ninety-nine'.

(f) *Silence.* Remember what has already been said on this subject. 'Whatever you say,' wrote St Augustine, 'say it in such a way that your hearer believes you, believing hopes, and hoping loves'. Every doctor should make these beautiful words his own.

Earlier on I suggested that 'optitechnique' should be made part of a doctor's training in symptomatology. There is even more reason for clinical 'logotechnique': the art of using both verbal psychotherapy and exploratory questioning when speaking to the patient. In the *Charmides* Plato wrote that 'fair speech' (*logos kalos*) was necessary to the perfection of the art of healing. In the preceding pages I have merely tried to apply this profound Platonic saying to the modern situation.

3 Besides looking at the patient and talking to him, the doctor lays his hands on his body in order to carry out the three classic operations of manual examination: percussion, palpation and ausculation. Text-books on physical examination explain how a doctor should carry out these techniques, and what discoveries they may lead to. I cannot embark on this subject, but shall go in some detail into the question of what part manual contact between examiner and patient

plays in the whole structure of the medical relationship.

Let us begin by studying the doctor's tactile experience. When he puts his hands on the patient's body, what does he gain from this contact besides certain information about the physical state of the body he is exploring? A person may touch another's body as if it were merely an 'object', or else think of it as the somatic reality of an individual 'persona'. In the first case, he notices various objective signs (hard or soft, smooth or rough, etc.), adjusts or alters the position of his hands in space, and experiences a feeling of pleasure (it might be called a caress-for-me) or displeasure regardless of the patient as a person. In the second, the doctor aware that what he is touching is human, adjusts or alters the position of his hands in space for personal reasons and, besides experiencing pleasure or displeasure, tries to make the other person experience it also (in the case of pleasure, the caress-for-the-other-person). It follows that palpation must be two things for the doctor: both an objective and cognitive operation, and, in a complementary manner, an interpersonal act of love, a true caress-for-the-other-person. There are two reasons for this. Since taction and palpation are nearly always disturbing, they must start as actual caresses, so that the patient will relax the defensive muscles of the area being explored. Secondly, an amorous contact, or caress, always gives the recipient comfort and support. Just as a look can be a haven, a hand can also be a haven, and this is what the doctor's hand should be. It is hardly necessary to say that aesthetic and moral delicacy are imperatively demanded.

And what about the patient's tactile experience? As a

Apparatus and instruments at the height of the Victorian era. They illustrate a report published in *The Graphic* of 30 July 1881, of an International Sanitary and Medical Exhibition.

complete human experience, not merely as a neuro-physiological process, what is the nature of the sensation of 'being touched'? Supposing that the person in question accepts the contact and does not rebel against it, there may be four components of his experience. First, an experience of self-assertion. More or less consciously a person who receives an amorous caress reaches an inner conclusion on the Cartesian model: 'I am being caressed, therefore I am not worthless'. Secondly, a sense of relaxation. By means of this sense of relaxation, skilful palpation can succeed (as Nacht says) "in giving a holiday to the adult man, who is unconsciously striving so hard to quiet the little boy crying inside him'. Kamala, the wolf-child of Midnapore, could only be truly comforted by being massaged by Mrs Singh.[9] Thirdly, a sense of comfort and company. Skilfully carried out, such a contact is consoling and provides encouragement and companionship, especially when the person touching is thought of by the person touched as outstandingly important and eminent. The ritual or magic formality of 'laying on of hands' is based on this psychological phenomenon. Fourthly, an experience of pleasure, generically felt as well-being and specifically modulated according to the area receiving the amorous contact.

Such – subject to the most fastidious moral discipline – should be the manual relation between doctor and patient. Besides 'optitechnique' and 'logotechnique', it is equally important that a doctor's education should include 'cheirotechnique' – or the art of using the hands.

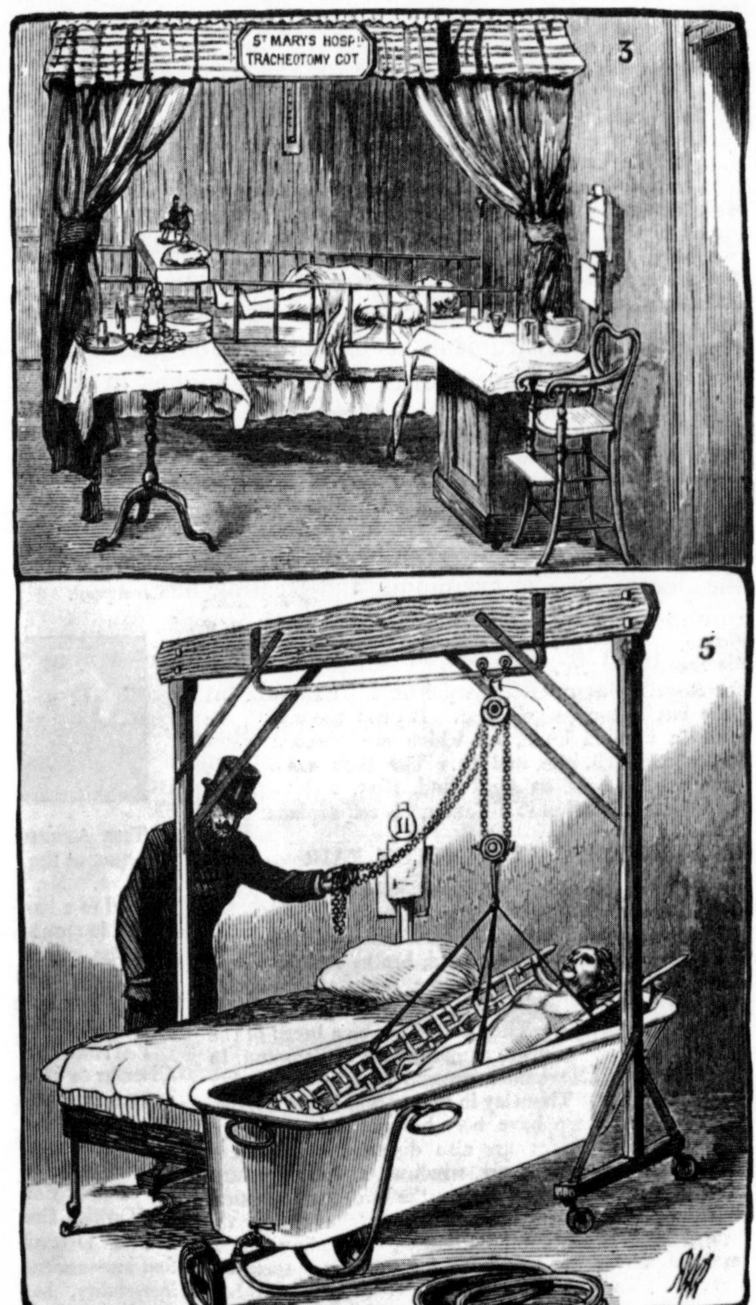
St MARYS HOSPl.
TRACHEOTOMY COT
3
5

4 Communication between doctor and patient is also (increasingly since the eighteenth century) a matter of instruments. The thermometer, stethoscope, sphygmomanometer, ophthalmoscope, X-ray apparatus, electrocardiogram, and a hundred other instruments act as indispensable aids. What is the significance of a medical instrument looked at in this light? It has several – three at least. First and foremost, it is a technical means of enlarging the doctor's facilities for diagnosis and therapy. Thus considered, the instrument fulfils the function, on the margin of his objective activities, of increasing the patient's confidence in medicine and hence in the doctor who is examining and treating him. There are quite a few patients who hand themselves over more confidently from the start to doctors and diagnosticians who have plenty of 'apparatus' at their disposal. So much so, that medicine in which doctors have been totally replaced by technical instruments often figures in modern Utopias (F. Paycha and others). The truth is that technical instruments can do *much* for both doctor and patient, but they cannot and should not do *everything*. Secondly, they are also symbolical objects. In other words they stand for or symbolise something else by reason of their shape (some time ago Ernest Jones gave a phallic interpretation of the stethoscope) or their function (for instance, the pressure on the arm by the arm-band of the sphygmomanometer). J. P. Valabrega dealt methodically with this symbolic element in his study of the medical relationship. Thirdly, and finally, it can be a separating wall between clinician and patient. Some invalids have a special need of personal contact with the doctor; and if he relies entirely on

instruments, or hides his own inadequate techniques behind them, the apparatus may cause failure of communication.

The emotional bond

Communication between doctor and patient fulfils a double function in respect of their mutual relation: on one hand it expresses the nature of the bond created between them by the conjunction of their respective aims; on the other, its reaction on this initial bond establishes its special and concrete psychological consistency. In the next paragraph we shall study the affective aspect of the link between therapist and patient, when the relationship is medically correct.

1 First let us look at the various cardinal forms of the emotional link between doctor and patient. Supposing that this link has been effectively established (and this does not always happen – think of the surgeon who operates on an unconscious patient and leaves his post-operative care to others), we know that correctly it may take three forms: medical comradeship, transference, and medical philia in the strict sense.

I call the bond between doctor and patient medical comradeship when both are working for the patient's health as a purely objective good, and dispensing with anything that could strictly be called 'personal' in diagnosis and treatment. When patients are of a certain sort – when they belong to the sociological and psychological type of Riesman's 'inner-directed man', and their lives are controlled by a moral imperative to be self-sufficient – medical treatment has usually to be based on a relation of affectionate comradeship. But even this medical comradeship sometimes develops beyond an individual line of conduct and becomes a political ideal. This happens when the individual has to adjust his whole life to the aims of the state. In such societies, health is good only insofar as it serves those aims, and the doctor is the official responsible for it. In principle, the totalitarian view of the medical relationship fits into this scheme. In treatment of the mentally sick, the Nazis showed with terrible clarity to what lengths a state could go when the health of its members was merely a 'public good'.

The case of the transference is very different. Earlier I quoted a short extract in which Freud first mentioned this phenomenon. Very early on in their careers as psychotherapists, both Breuer and Freud noticed in their patients unequivocal signs of erotic feeling for the person of their doctor. Breuer was so disturbed by this that he broke off treatment, and abandoned the new technique of psychoanalysis for ever. Freud, however, realised the psychological significance of the phenomenon, and discovered how to make it into one of the most important foundation-stones of psychoanalytical therapy. The transference presupposed the patient's profound confidence in the doctor, and a good observer can discover it, says Freud, in every medical activity entailing close cooperation with the patient and tending to modify his psychological state. Operating on the situation created by psychoanalysis, three elements in combination – interest, the doctor's active sympathy and his personal authority – always give rise to the phenomenon of transference. The doctor then becomes the illuminator of the patient's consciousness, master of his life, and to some extent confessor of his intimate problems. Later on Freud was to describe the 'counter-transference' or reciprocal transference, in which the transference situation is reflected in the therapist's psyche and projected on to the personality of the patient.

In my view, medical philia is different from both medical comradeship and transference. Let us imagine the relationship between a chronic invalid and his doctor. In this case the physician visits his patient frequently; if he is a really good doctor he will know all about the invalid's life, receive his confidences, invent plans for improving his existence and help him realise them, and enter sympathetically into his feelings about his illness and his hopes of new health; in a word, he will establish a truly affectionate relation with him, a specifically 'medical' philia which we will presently clarify.

2 We must now examine the mutual relation between these three cardinal forms of the bond between doctor and patient. Three questions seem to emerge.

(a) *Is it possible for there to be a good medical comradeship which yet has no element of true friendship?* Personally, I do not think so. The restoration of health the doctor is striving for is first and foremost for the benefit of the patient, and must surely be seen as such by any practitioner whose mind is not closed to everything but obstinate political fanaticism. Even if the doctor holds the doctrinaire belief that his bond with his patient can and should be nothing more than medical comradeship, human nature is such that it is bound to make the relationship to some extent 'friendly': the doctor is using his technical skill for the patient's benefit – chiefly, if not entirely – and the patient trusts the man who has put his knowledge and goodwill at his disposal.

(b) *What is the relation between medical philia and the transference?* The reality and theory of the transference was a very frequent theme of Freud's later researches; the bibliography on the subject is enormous, and I cannot therefore go into it in detail here. I must confine myself to answering the previous question briefly.

On one side we have a transference relation between a neurotic patient and his analyst. On the other, we have a medical philia between someone suffering from heart disease and the clinician who is treating him. Is medical philia perhaps a sublimated form of the minimal transference that was set up between doctor and patient at the outset of their relation? Is the transference perhaps the instinctive emotional response of an individual human being when philia has become sufficiently intense in him? Did not Plato say that when philia grew sufficiently ardent it became *erôs,* and Aristotle that *erôs* was an exaggerated form of philia? I will tabulate my replies in the following four points:

First, in their pure forms, transference and philia are two qualitatively different sorts of interhuman link. The transference is above all an instinctive phenomenon, and therefore – as a closer analysis will show – has a generic reality as its object. Whereas philia is a personal phenomenon, and its object is the unique and untransferable personality of the friend. This seems to me directly applicable to the medical relationship.

Secondly, although essentially different, both transference and philia are solidly based on interhuman relationships, but since one or the other element usually predominates, relations between individuals may be preponderantly 'friendly' or 'transferential'.

Thirdly, when a preponderantly friendly relationship becomes more intense, the transference phenomena – hitherto slight – grow stronger and more apparent. This is why Christian asceticism is usually suspicious of intensified 'personal friendships'.

Fourthly, when a preponderantly transferential relationship is purified and becomes personal, its aim ceases to be an 'object' and becomes a 'subject'; more precisely, 'an individual'. This is what happens when the psychotherapist is skilful enough to turn the phenomena of transference and counter-transference to account.

(c) *What is the true nature of medical philia?* How does philia become 'medical'? The specific character of the invalid's friendship for the doctor is *trust*. The patient confidently expects that the doctor will help him to regain his health, although this hope always contains a tiny thread of fear, lest his illness should 'take a bad turn', or the doctor fail to 'hit the mark'. The invalid's trust takes verbal form in confidences. When the relationship is correct the patient talks confidentially to the doctor; he is not merely confiding in his doctor as such, but also – and perhaps above all – in the unique individual his doctor happens to be.

Benevolence, an eighteenth-century view after Marillier.

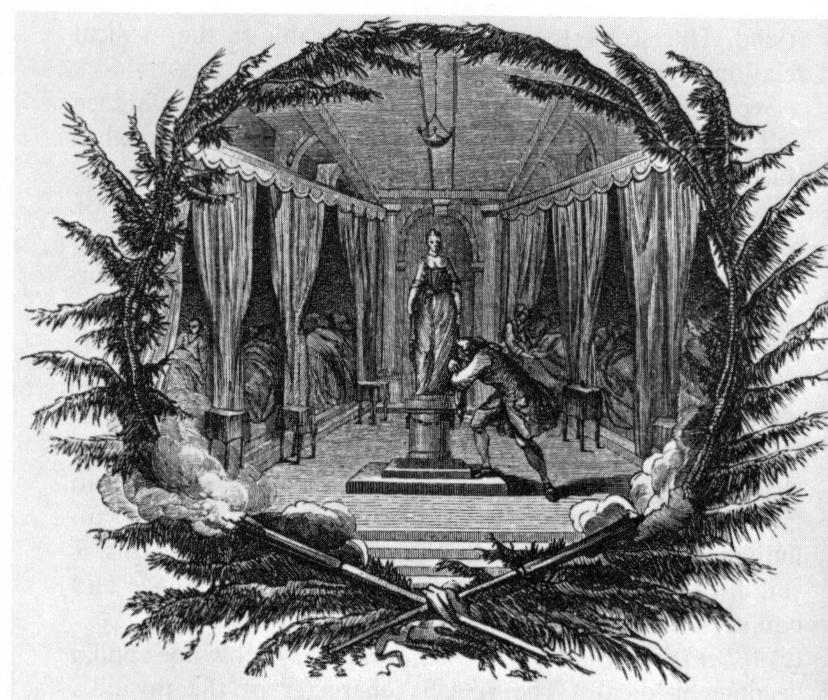

Fig. 157. — La statue de la Bienfaisance, érigée dans un hôpital.
(Composition allégorique d'après Marillier.)

The doctor's friendship for the patient should consist above all in a desire to give effective technical help – *benevolence* conceived and realised in technical terms. The patient's health is of value to the doctor, otherwise he would not labour to restore it; but it also is of value to the patient himself. And so, although the doctor's activity necessarily has technical and transferential ingredients, it is 'personalised' – and so to speak 'made friendly' – by explicit reference to the personality of the patient.

Plato called medicine 'the science of what pertains to the love of the body'. Science, technique and love are combined in one way or another in the acitivity of a good doctor. But what is that love? I would say that medical treatment ought to be at the same time *erôs, agapê* and philia. Like every other vocation, the vocation of healing is *erôs:* love of its own perfection and the perfection of the world in which the vocation is realised. But it must be realised; and when this happens the direct contact of the healer with the reality in which his vocation is exercised changes *erôs* into *agapê,* and converts it into an effusion of love. It is thus that the artist, the sage and the politician love the world through their vocations. However, there are certain vocations that happen to have other people as their direct object; first and foremost among them come medicine and teaching. What happens when one of these vocations is put into practice? It will obviously end by being expressed in acts of philia – a philia more or less harmoniously blended with the special technical activity entailed by the character of the vocation itself: medical philia in the case of the therapist and educative philia in that of the teacher. That is why I said before that a therapist's activity was at the same time *erôs, agapê* and philia, love as desire, love outgoing, and friendship.

3 Up to the present I have only referred to the correct forms of the emotional link between doctor and patient. This is not an unattainable ideal. But it must be recognised that in actual medical treatment corrupt or incorrect practices do occur, and something must be said about them.

The medical relation may be incorrect in the first place because of excess or defect in the emotional content of the friendly bond. Typical examples of such incorrectness are: morbid intensification of the phenomena of transference and counter-transference, and the simultaneous technical or moral inability of the doctor to free them from the dominion of the 'id'; excessive coldness on the doctor's part, emphasising his scientific or official role, when the patient consciously or unconsciously demands to be treated as something more than the 'object' of a technical operation; the temptation for a doctor to transform his technical superiority over the patient into the sort of conduct Balint has described as 'the apostolic function', namely to imply that the cure cannot be complete unless the doctor succeeds in converting his patient to his own vision of an ideal world; mutual seduction, not of a sexual nature, into which both doctor and patient are sometimes drawn – this consists in the doctor being excessively credulous of what his adulatory patient tells him about his sufferings, while the patient on his side openly flatters the doctor's complacency and vanity (Balint).

The medical relation can also become corrupt when the feeling linking therapist and patient is not a friendly one in the broadest sense of the word, or if it is, when it is enveloped and dominated by some other emotion. The two commonest examples of this are (in the doctor) an excessive desire to make money, so that 'philia' becomes merely 'tactical amiability', and (in the patient) too great a sense of his own rights, both in regard to the doctor himself, whom he sees merely as a salesman of diagnosis and therapy, and in regard to society and its obligations to provide medical care, represented in his eyes by the therapist.

Whether the reader is a doctor, an invalid, or a possible invalid, his knowledge of the world he lives in will make it easy for him to fill in this schematic outline with palpitating life.

The cognitive element

The task of diagnosis begins for the doctor as soon as he meets his patient. To see a sick man is to start diagnosing him. From a purely formal point of view, diagnosis consists in studying what has been offered him of the patient's previous experiences and present state, framing a hypothesis which appears to explain them, and attempting to confirm this hypothesis by definite explorative measures, substituted by others if confirmation is not forthcoming and continuing in this manner until he gains a sufficient knowledge of his patient to understand fully all the facts about him that experience has provided. This is the method, as a Hippocratic physician would describe it.

The military hospital at Fortress Monroe during the American Civil War. As most battle cases require surgery, accurate diagnosis is often self-evident, though in this century, and particularly since World War Two, more attention is given to general stress factors. These often date from a patient's peace-time childhood, and are thus highly individual.

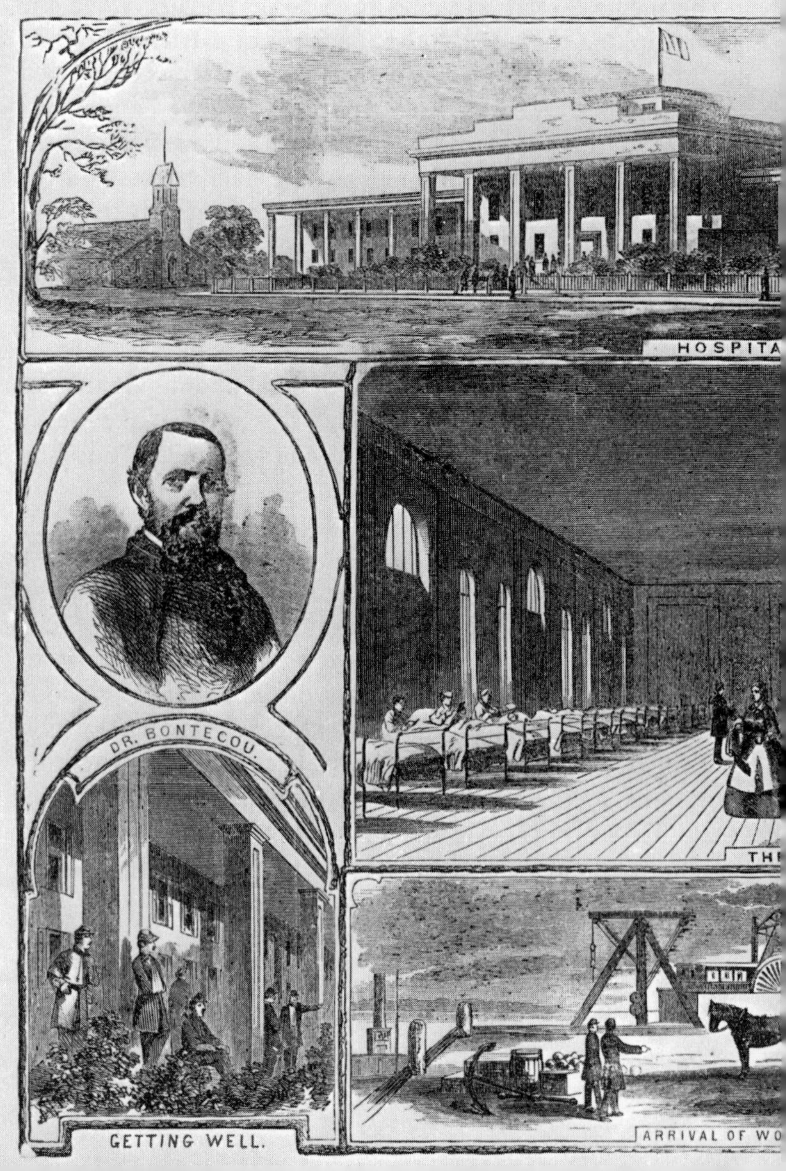

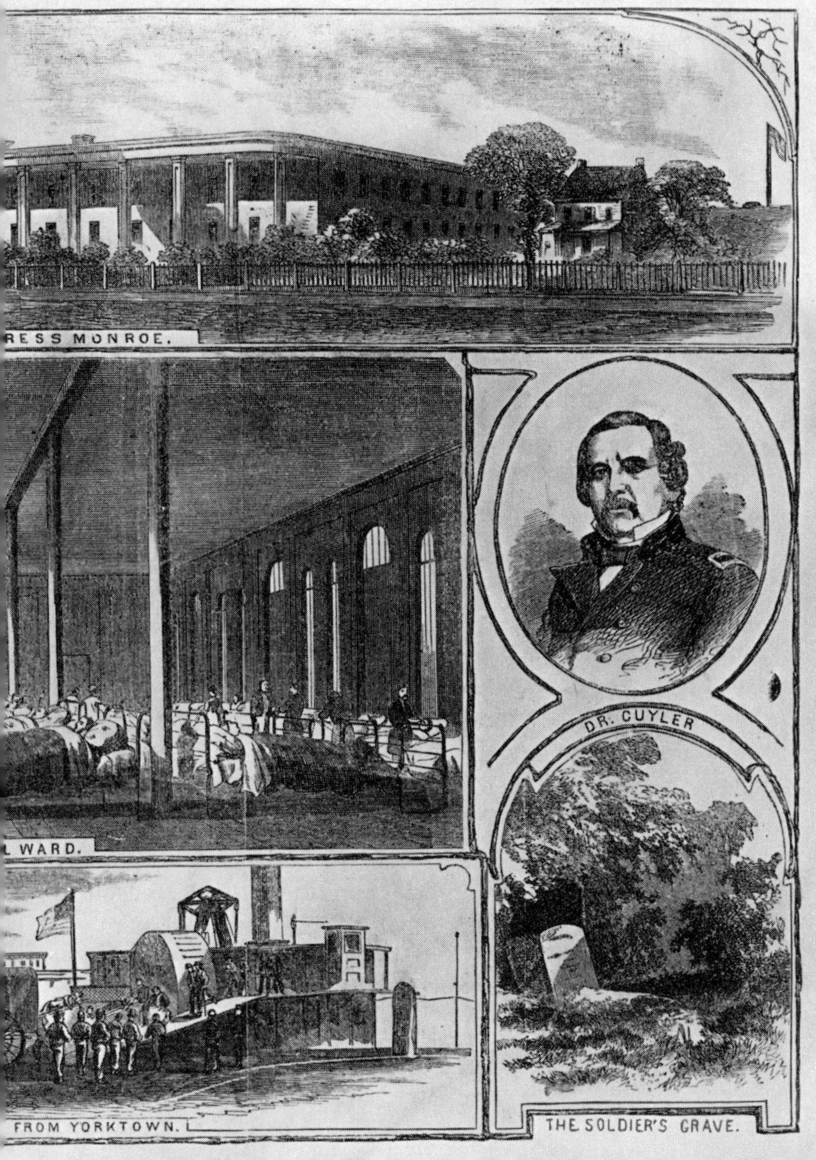
RESS MONROE.
DR. CUYLER
WARD.
FROM YORKTOWN.
THE SOLDIER'S GRAVE.

However, this formal scheme can be interpreted in various different ways. What does clinical experience consist in, technically speaking? By asking a sufferer from stomach ulcers, or an asthmatic, how he gets on with the other members of his family, does the doctor acquire scientifically significant clinical experience, or merely satisfy his curiosity, which as Claude Bernard would say 'has nothing to do with science'? Obviously one must distinguish carefully between the different methods of diagnosis. I shall reduce them to two: one, which I shall call 'classical' or 'scientifico-natural' and the other to which I shall give the name of 'integral' or 'scientifico-personal'.

The scientifico-natural concept of diagnosis is based on three activities: objectivation (when the diagnosis gives a name to an actual objective disorder in the patient, such as a lung cavity or hyperglycaemia), specification (as pulmonary tuberculosis or diabetes) and induction (the diagnostic verdict resulting from an inductive process of the mind). But a careful examination of the facts shows that the diagnosis cannot be *only* specific and *only* objective, because the patient's attitude to his doctor and to his own illness modifies the clinical picture to some extent, and because the doctor's own point of view – that of an 'ego' which may be *sapiens, cupiens, fungens* or *adiuvans* (see page 107) – intervenes to some extent in the exploratory apprehension and mental configuration of what is observed. When the doctor makes a diagnosis, he does not and cannot confine himself to objectifying and specifying what he finds in his patient. To sum up, diagnosis always involves something more than saying (truthfully) 'this man is suffering from diabetes'.

The scientifico-personal concept of diagnosis is more ambitious, and attempts to take into consideration the whole somatic, psychological and personal state of the patient, that is to say his entire individual and social reality. As we know, this entails the twofold and complementary task of personalising the findings reached by somatic and psychological observation of the invalid, and objectifying as far as possible those obtained from co-operation in the patient's personal reaction to his own illness.

Although the doctor may not be aware of the fact, the diagnosis may be directed as follows:

General diagnosis, or the reply to the question 'Is this man really and truly ill?'. In most cases an affirmative reply will be given in objective terms (coma, haemorrhage, bloated features, jaundice, etc.); but an observant clinician will have to decide whether the patient's personal attitude to his own illness (complaints, depression, etc.) is really and truly justified by the disease itself, and this entails mental objectivity and co-operation on his part. This will be even more necessary when the reply to this question involves the possibility of neurosis or malingering.

Specific diagnosis, or an adequate reply to the question 'What special disease is this man suffering from?'. The very reality of the 'morbid condition' means that the diagnosis must be objective and not personal. The methods described in textbooks on symptomatology are generally used, although it is always possible to be presented with the subtle problem of the patient's personal reaction to suffering from 'this disease' and not 'the other'.

Individual diagnosis, or the scientific understanding of what is strictly personal to the case under observation. It is often said that there are no diseases, only patients. It would be better to say: 'There are diseases, and patients suffering from them,' because the actual illness is almost invariably the result of the individualisation of a specific disease. How, then does this individualisation of the illness take place? Scientifico-natural pathology replies with the concept – actually a medieval one: the 'principle of individualisation' as *materia signata quantitate* – of the quantitative individualisation of illness; the amount and duration of hyperglycaemia after a load of glucose, the degree of polyuria and emaciation, etc., give individuality to Mr X's diabetes. More satisfactory is the concept of qualitative individualisation, according to which a case is made individual by the complete clinical picture (of specific and individual symptoms, and their mutual relationship in space and time). But without denying the partial validity of either criterion, it is plain that the only personal individualisation of the case can be integral: that is to say, methodical and scientific reference of all the observed facts to the person of the patient. Here we are faced with three main questions: First, the biographical occasion, or *kairos,* of the onset of the disease. Why did it appear when it did in the patient's life and not at another time? Secondly, the peculiar configuration of the picture of the symptoms. What part was played in it by the individuality of the patient?

Thirdly, personal attitude. How did the patient's personality 'adopt' or reject his illness? Fourthly, personal creativity. To what extent and in what manner – consciously or unconsciously – is the patient the creator of his own clinical picture? To what degree is he the 'agent' of his illness as well as the 'patient'?

Thus conceived, the disease process is no longer merely 'matter individually marked by quantity' (*materia quantitate signata*), it is 'quantitative matter determined by constitution, creation and interpretation' (*materia constitutione, creatione et interpretatione quantitative signata*); in no other way can the human and personal character of an individual case be understood. And the clinician can only achieve this by combining four mental activities: objectivation (methodical study of the somatic and psychological state of the patient as an object of scientific knowledge and technical manipulation), induction (necessary in order to diagnose the specific disease), interpretation (applied both to observed facts concerning the patient and to his own personal interpretation of his illness), and co-operation (directed towards the intimate behaviour of the invalid as patient, co-actor and co-author of the diseased condition).

A diagnostic verdict is not and never has been the result of a cognitive encounter between the doctor's 'pure reason' and the patient's 'purely external and objective state', but it is the cognitive expression of the continuous link that has existed between them since they first met in their present capacities. Without a true 'medical philia' in the sense I have already given this expression, how could the doctor's diagnosis be 'personal' as well as objective and specific?

The operative element

Once the treatment has begun, the doctor-patient relationship reaches its culminating point. What is the essence of medical treatment? As with diagnosis, this question can be given two answers: one is 'classical' or 'scientifico-natural', the other 'integral' or 'scientifico-personal'.

The scientifico-natural concept of treatment depends upon three principles. First, the therapeutic effect of the remedy must be objectively and experimentally verified, preferably by a controlled trial. Secondly, it must be applied as a result of clinically and scientifically valid indications. Thirdly, the remedy must be correctly administered. A treatment which fulfils these three conditions must in principle be effective.

It would be both unjust and foolish to close one's eyes to great and effective results obtained as a result of this concept of therapy; but no less unjust and foolish to deny that medical treatment does not consist in this alone – a realisation that owes much in recent years to Wolf and other students of the 'Placebo' effect – the clinical response to treatments that are in themselves ineffective. There are five aspects of this. First, treatment begins before it has been formally embarked upon. Ernst von Leyden used to tell his pupils 'A doctor starts treating his patient when he shakes hands with him'. Secondly, the patient usually takes part in his own treatment; not only by passively carrying out the doctor's suggestions, but also deliberately, because he usually *knows* something about the treatment of illness. Thirdly, throughout his dealings with the patient, the doctor – who is a sort of medicine in himself

(Maeder, Balint) – is having a favourable or unfavourable effect on the disease. Fourthly, the therapy prescribed varies considerably according to the personality of the doctor; it is sufficient to remember that there are doctors who are 'always prescribing' and others who 'prescribe very seldom'. Fifthly, in every society, the group or class to which the patient belongs has an effect on the form and content of his treatment.

In order to understand what really happens, we must therefore make use of a scientifico-personal concept of medical treatment, and consider respectively two typical cases: treatment of acute and of chronic illness.

In acute illness, if effective therapy is available the treatment will coincide entirely or almost entirely with that dictated by the scientifico-natural principles already described. For example, let us suppose a doctor is faced with a patient suffering from a prefebrile malarial shivering fit. Without exchanging a single word, he immediately suspects the cause of what he sees, tests his hypothesis by an examination of the patient's blood, prescribes the proper remedy and completely cures his trouble. There is no question about this. Nor is there any question that, as we have known since Plato's day, the effectiveness of remedies is increased by the therapist's suggestive power and support. For this reason, a proper 'personal' relation between doctor and patient is therapeutically desirable even in acute illness.

The case of chronic illness is very different. Here the patient has to build his life in some way around his sufferings, and this entails a different approach to the aim, structure and shape of the treatment.

Of course the aim of medical treatment must always be the recovery of health. But there are times when neither doctor nor patient can count on this, and others when recuperation is problematical, and calls for very prolonged treatment. What should be the immediate aim of therapy in these two cases? The patient should undoubtedly lead the best possible life compatible with treating the illness. The doctor must therefore invent a *bios,* or way of life, in which the limitations imposed by illness and the possibilities it still allows are combined to the best possible advantage. It is no exaggeration to say that the therapist needs to be both a novelist and a sculptor in regard to this other person's life: a novelist because he invents a life for the patient, and a sculptor because he realises his invention and uses his art to modify the patient's nature and teach him how to live.

Something of the same sort can be said of the internal aspects of the treatment. What roles do doctor, remedy and patient play here? As the inventor and sculptor of the patient's *vita nuova,* the doctor is his comrade, teacher and friend – a man who is medically his friend because therapy involves the patient's trust (without which the invention of the 'possible personality' would be impossible) and also his benevolent co-operation in personal activity. The remedy now reaches its maximum complexity, for treatment of a chronic illness often calls upon all the therapeutic resources of modern medicine. Is it possible for the patient to accept the biological effect of these remedies in a purely passive manner? Obviously not: he must have a genuine desire to get well and to co-operate with the doctor, both by willingly accepting the suggested regime – 'obey your doctor and you start getting well', wrote Marañon – and by interpreting the advice he is given in his own personal way.

All this is impossible when the treatment is not given form by a genuinely friendly relationship, particularly if the link between therapist and patient is not a strictly 'interpersonal' one. A doctor by vocation will be friend to his patients, and especially when they are chronically ill. In such cases the treatment is the active manifestation of medical philia.[10]

The ethical element

Like all truly human behaviour, the relation between doctor and patient has an ethical aspect for each of them. Unlike animals, whose instincts help them to 'adapt' to their environment, man is constantly having to use his freedom and intelligence to adapt his behaviour to his situation; in this way 'adaptation' becomes 'justification' (Zubiri), and therefore moral (or immoral) behaviour. This happens to both doctor and patient in their relationship. In the doctor's case, his personal acceptance of his own status as a doctor, the way he receives his patient and carries out different exploratory and therapeutic operations, and the fixing of a fee, are actions that can be morally or immorally performed. And the same can be said, in the patient's case, of the 'personal' way he takes his own illness, and his conduct to the doctor attending him.

The doctor's duties to a sick man consist simply in carrying out the golden rule of the art of healing: working for the good of the patient. But what is the patient's good, strictly speaking? What ought it to consist in, in a given case? Can the good of an individual be achieved without conflict? While they by no means exhaust the theme, the following are the chief 'fields of conflict' in which the ethical nature of his relation to the patient are revealed to the doctor:

First, *the possible conflict between the individual and society*. Society insists that the invalid – a head of state, perhaps, or a general during a military campaign – must return immediately to his social obligations, whereas the sick man does not want to resume work until he feels completely and solidly restored to health. Another possibility: for certain reasons the state or society does not want the invalid to recover, yet he is clamouring to be cured quickly. What should the doctor do in these two cases?

Secondly, *the conflict between objective considerations and the patient's personal interests*. Failure to use psychotherapy, out of negligence or haste, may in some cases be as ethically serious a piece of carelessness as not to examine the responses of the pupil to light would be in another case.

Thirdly, *the conflict between declaring or concealing the illness*. The diagnostic verdict is completed when the doctor communicates it to the patient. But how far should he go in telling the patient about his illness?

Fourthly, *the conflict between the need to be assiduous and the need to be detached*. Medical treatment is not entirely satisfactory without some degree of assiduity; nor yet without some detachment.

Fifthly, *the conflict between 'can' and 'ought'*. Technique consists as much in 'knowing how something should be done' as in 'being able to do it'. A modern doctor can do much technically for human nature. In some cases the question arises: ought he to do all he can?

Sixthly, *the conflict between desire for the highest fee and the obligation to ask a just fee*. This occurs rather more frequently when the fee is freely agreed upon by doctor and patient between themselves.

Although the state of being ill exempts the sick man from some social obligations, he still has obligations to his doctor. The three chief ones are: loyalty, confidence and detachment. Loyalty will induce him to tell his doctor everything bearing on his illness. Of course confidence cannot be produced at will; but the patient can and should cultivate it in himself. Inconstancy in choice of a doctor and in forming a bond with him is very damaging. Finally, detachment – affectionate detachment – will prevent confidence and friendship turning a useful transference into a morbid one.

Modified and given roots by their respective beliefs as to the ultimate meaning of life, these in my view are the principal obligations of doctor and patient in their mutual relationship.

Social aspects of the medical relationship

'When I see a patient, he and I are on a desert island', Schweninger, one of the most eminent clinicians in Bismarck's Berlin, used often to say. Nothing could be more representative of the individualism of the last century, nor could anything be more false. Whether they know it or not, doctor and patient are all the time affected by the society they belong to, and modern medicine recognises this fact. Indeed, during the last few decades a new branch of medicine, social medicine, has emerged; it is not and cannot be the whole of medicine but it is an essential part.

This means that much of what the previous pages contain is in some sense a conventional and systematic abstraction, because the doctor-patient relationship is in its very essence social. We will go on to study in turn the social element in individual illness, the social status of the doctor as such, and the social aspect of the relation between him and his patient.

1 Except for the intimate experiences it involves, everything to do with illness has an undoubted social character: its cause, the way it is endured, the pattern of the symptomatic picture.

Let us consider the *causa morbi*. As Galen long ago taught, it is made up of elements that are external or primitive (poison, bacteria, trauma, emotion, etc.,) internal and dispositional (individual susceptibility), and direct and immediate (the principal anatomo-physiological changes produced by the two previous ingredients and combined with them). How can we disregard the important part played by society in the two first? The penetration of the patient's body by disease-bearing bacteria or poison, the action upon it of a mechanical or emotional trauma, and the part of the body affected – everything in fact that makes up the external cause of the illness – is to some extent socially determined. However strange it may appear at first sight, this includes even the genesis of neoplasms. The most recent statistical investigations (in the United States, Britain, Germany, Norway, South Africa and Indonesia) have very clearly shown that there is a relation between the incidence of malignant tumours and social class: cancer of the stomach, lung and the neck of the uterus are more frequent among the poorer classes; cancer of the colon, rectum and breast among the rich. Whatever the mechanism, there is a social factor in the genesis and localisation of cancer. The same can be said of the three factors (genetic, developmental and educational) that make up the dispositional cause. For example, is not ancestry a social as well as a genetic concept? In the developmental aspect of the individual constitution – and therefore of the individual susceptibility – I include the effect of the double gestation, uterine and social, which every human being undergoes.* The zoologist Portman has made a brilliant study of the immaturity of our species at birth, and has suggested giving the name of 'social uterus' to the protective and formative environment that surrounds a child during the first months of its extra-uterine existence, in which the mother or her substitute plays far the most important part. An immense amount of biological, psychological and clinical research (by Spitz, Silvia Brody, Sullivan, Bowlby, Rof Carballo, etc.) has shown how very important this 'social uterus' is in the individual's somatic and psychological development, in the acquisition of the culture patterns of the group he belongs to (Ruth Benedict, Margaret Mead) and in the development of his various path-

* This is discussed at length in Philippe Muller's *The Tasks of Childhood* (World University Library).

Pasteur and some of his patients who suffered from hydrophobia. Social and genetic influences can create a 'dispositional cause' for certain diseases.

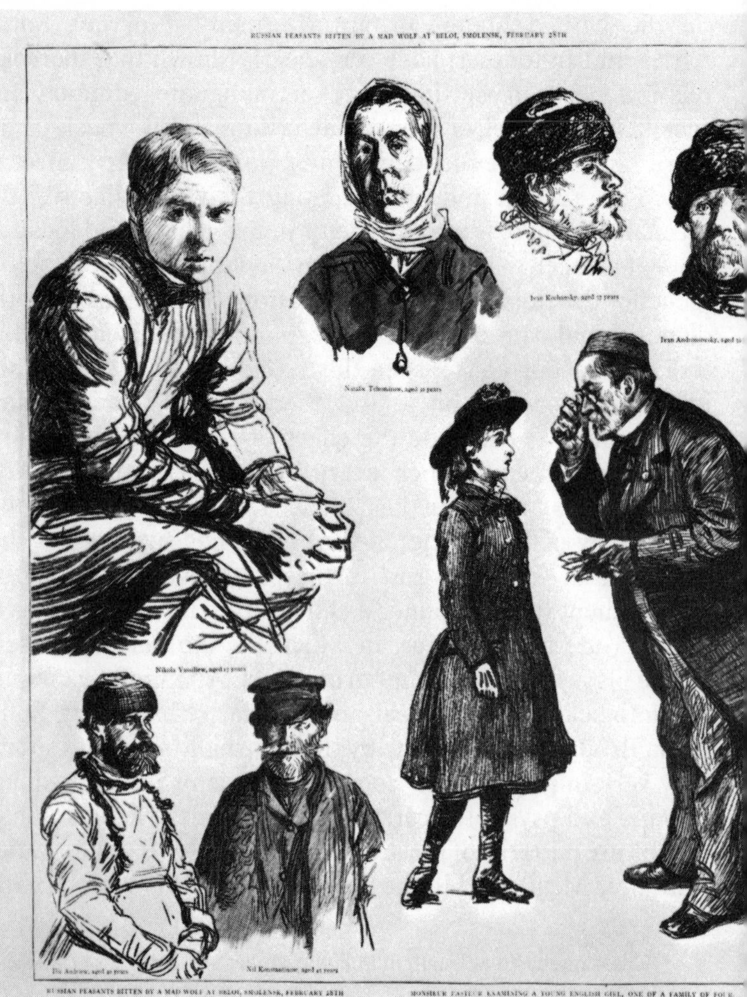

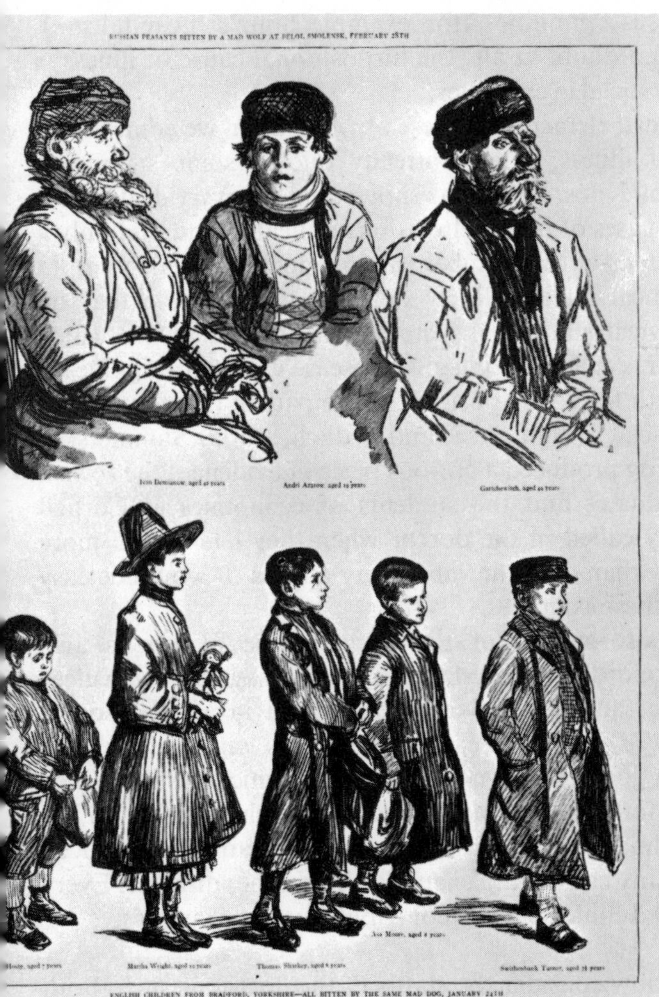
RUSSIAN PEASANTS BITTEN BY A MAD WOLF AT BELOI, SMOLENSK, FEBRUARY 28TH
ENGLISH CHILDREN FROM BRADFORD, YORKSHIRE—ALL BITTEN BY THE SAME MAD DOG, JANUARY 24TH

ological susceptibilities (for example Spitz's 'hospitalism'). There is no doubt at all: the dispositional cause of illness is markedly social in character.

The social element is no less obvious when we come to the feeling of illness. I have already quoted some significant findings by Koos. Braun has shown that for every death there are 1,200 cases of trivial alterations of health, and that only a few hundreds of this number call in a doctor. The decision to take medical advice clearly depends to a large extent on psychological and social factors. The frequency with which the doctor is called in for a given disease varies to a significant degree with the social position of the patient (Freedman and Hollingshead, Hollingshead and Redlich, Stopp). Summerskill and Darling produced a curious piece of evidence: the Jewish undergraduates and the students of economics at Cornell University called in the doctor when they had a cold more frequently than did other university groups. It would be easy to add to these examples.

The conformation of the symptomatic picture is also socially conditioned. As Marañon used to say, 'Stomach ulcer is not the same disease in a reaper and in a professor of philosophy'. The subject of 'symptoms and society' has received a good deal of notice in recent clinical research. The work of Hollingshead and Redlich on psychiatric disease has become almost a classic; Ruesch and Bowman have produced a great many convincing examples from other diseases. Every experienced clinician could contribute further examples.

2 Let us now consider the status of the doctor as such. Both

the standard of his technical training and his manner of practising his profession essentially depend on the social group to which he belongs. Clinical practice in fact depends on: (a) The physician's economico-social outlook: some doctors have a capitalist and bourgeois outlook and others a socialist and proletarian one, and this influences their style of practice. (b) His reason for practising medicine. It will be remembered that the four main ones are desire to help, gain, search for knowledge, and a sense of official duty. (c) The social circumstances in which help is given to the sick. Some doctors are free, others are bound by contract, others function as officials, or as part of a socialist system; medical care can be provided in hospital, or at home, in private or public consulting-rooms. It is clear that there is a different way of establishing relations with the patient corresponding to each of these types of practice.

3 There is nothing surprising, therefore, in attributing a social character to the relation between doctor and patient. Although it is basically an interpersonal quasi-diadic link, it must essentially be seen within a social frame of reference which indeed determines it.

From a sociological point of view, what does the doctor-patient relationship consist in? The sociologist Talcott Parsons tells us that each individual in a given social unit is connected with the rest by a great many interacting relationships, and his function in the whole can be described by defining the position he occupies in that society (his *status*), and the part he plays in that position (his *role*). Now each role is

'Institutionalised expectations' define the role that society asks both doctor and patient to play. In a complex, partially modernised society, this role will be variable and will call for flexibility. A visit to a western-trained doctor may be followed by one to a native practitioner.

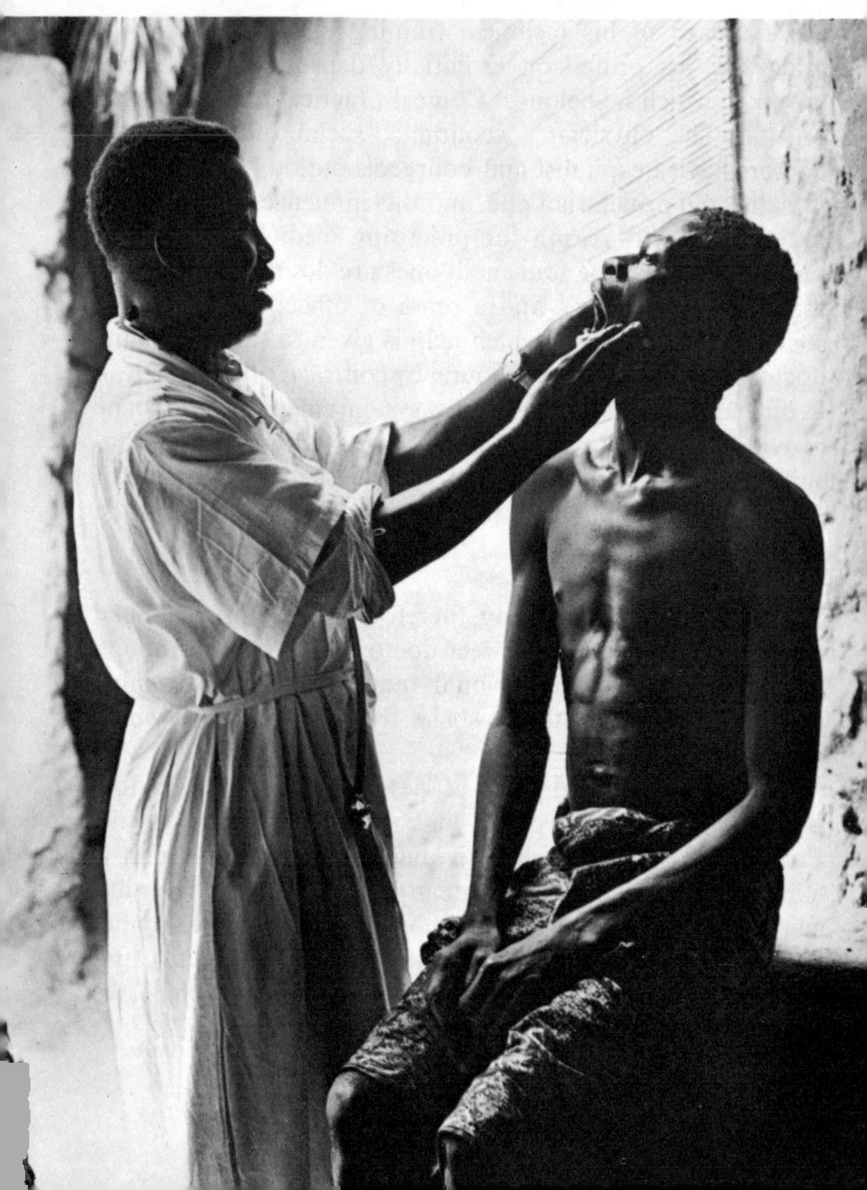

determined by the 'institutionalised expectations' appropriate to it – in other words, what is expected of the holder of the position by the social system in question. Parsons classifies the institutionalised expectations belonging to the role of the invalid in the civilised society of today as follows: (a) While he is ill, the patient is free from the social obligations entailed in the work he does when he is well. (b) However much he tries, the sick man cannot help being ill. As an invalid he is therefore exempt from his social responsibilities. (c) The patient must 'want to get well'. (d) The patient must ask for medical aid, and co-operate with the doctor who provides it. Society has reciprocal expectations of the doctor. If the occasion arises, he must help to free the patient from his social responsibilities (this is the purpose of 'medical certificates'), he must accept the patient's social irresponsibility, welcome his desire to get well, collaborate with him technically in the task of a cure, and refuse to allow him to use his illness to gain antisocial advantages.[11]

This is not the place to study the reception – favourable on the whole – given by the medical profession to Parsons' sociological scheme. According to his views the medical relation is essentially the result of mutual interaction between the doctor's and the patient's institutionalised expectations. If these correspond with those of the society they belong to, the relationship between them will be sociologically correct; if not, it will become a source of social conflict and discord. It would not seem difficult to establish a sociological typology of the faulty forms of the medical relation, based on the way doctor and patient realise their respective social obligations.

The sociology of the medical relation should also be studied 'from inside' – not only from the viewpoint of society but from that of the bipersonal unit made up of doctor and patient. Whether we call them 'affective-vegetative communication' like Von Ditfurth, or 'affective texture', like Rof Carballo, the connections with other people that are set up in the first days of extra-uterine life are necessary, as I have already observed, to the proper development of the human individual. When this has been defective or abnormal, it may cause emotional illness or perhaps even such diseases as pulmonary tuberculosis or gastric ulcer. And the protective, or as René Spitz calls it the 'diatrophic' part played by the patient's relation to his doctor, especially in cases of chronic illness or neurosis, can only be fully understood by a careful social analysis of his life history.

Conditioned 'from outside' (by society) and 'from inside' (through its bipersonal and quasi-diadic aspect), the medical relation is in itself a social one. Everyone can confirm this from his own experience of its different phases: the first meeting between doctor and patient, clinical examination, formation of an affective bond, diagnosis and treatment. Besides unavoidable 'personal' considerations, there are powerful 'social' ones affecting this relation, and its special character is determined by them both combined. I invite the reader to carry out the mental exercise of establishing the various typical forms of the medical relation, or – inversely – considering a special case and analysing it systematically in the light of my thesis. Perhaps a synopsis of the principal motives conditioning the form taken by the doctor-patient relationship may be helpful.

A ward in St Bartholomew's Hospital, London *c.* 1890.

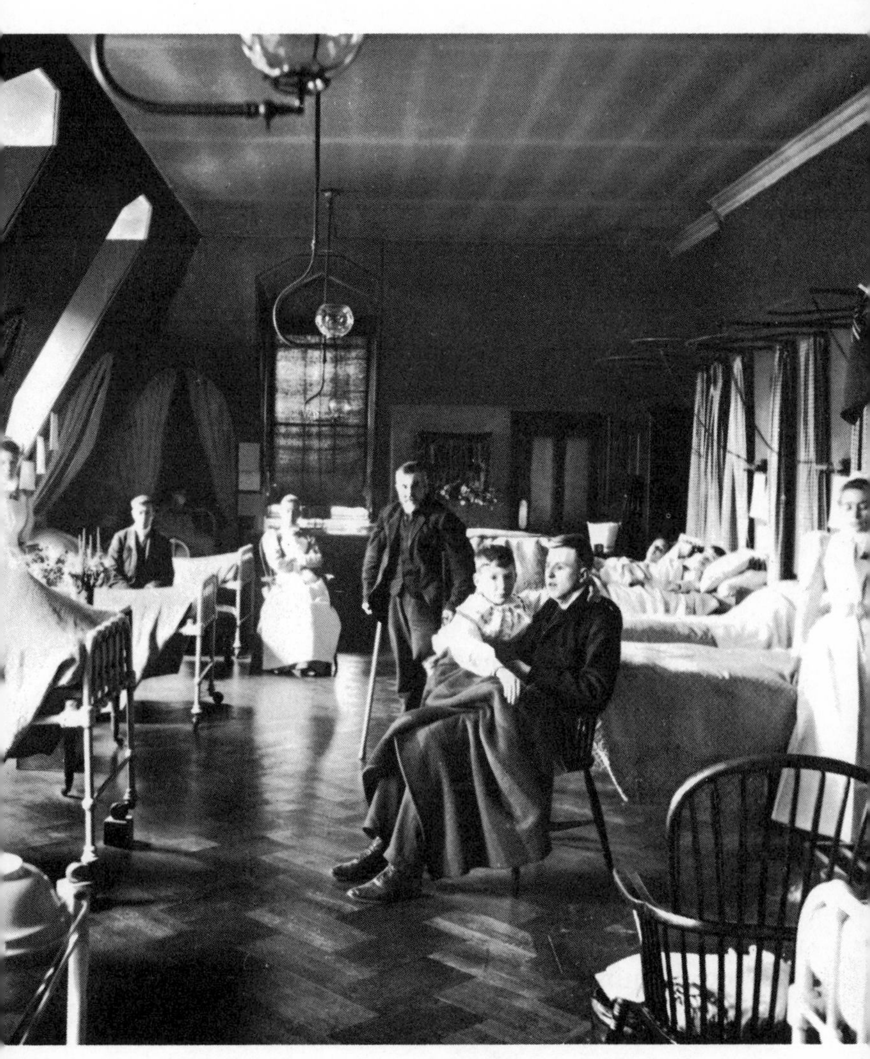

Personal motives

On the patient's part

1 What he is seeking and hoping for in his relation with this doctor.
2 What doctor he consults.
3 How he is aware of being ill.
4 How he has responded to his illness.
5 His attitude to medicine.
6 His attitude to the doctor as a person.

On the doctor's part

1 Adequacy of technique, and subjective awareness of it (confidence in himself as a doctor, or lack of it).
2 Dominant interest in his professional practice (scientific knowledge, financial gain, public function or desire to help the sick).
3 Personal considerations (temperamental and ethical).
4 Attitude towards the patient (how much he is a 'case' and how much a 'person').

Social motives

Relating to the patient

1 Motives for 'calling in the doctor' (role of society and of other people).
2 Social motives for feeling ill.
3 Social motives in response to illness.

Relating to the doctor

1 Technical training.
2 Social outlook.
3 Social aspect of his professional practice.

Relating to the medical relation itself

1 Social framework in which it takes place.
2 Institutionalised expectations of the social setting.
3 Social component in the quasi-diadic relation between doctor and patient.

6 The relationship today

In the preceding pages I have propounded a theory of the doctor-patient relation which seems to me in accord with modern medical thought and practice. I propose to devote my last chapter to a complementary study of the real nature of this relationship in modern society; but we must first take up the historical account broken off at the end of the Part 1, and study the different forms of the twentieth-century response to that rebellion of the subject which took place in the second half of the nineteenth.

The clinical aspect

Let us first look at the clinical aspect of that response. Against what was the rebellion directed? Against a society which largely ignored the real nature and worth of every man, regardless of his social position; and against an excessively objective and materialistic treatment of those who sought medical care. Current therapeutic methods, and the strong and universal belief in the technical possibilities of natural science, were not enough to deal with this very old and yet new manner of falling ill, and this led to the special character of the clinical response. Different schools of thought and even more varied personal standpoints (the names of Freud, Adler, Jung, Stekel, Dubois and Schultz speak for themselves) have helped doctors to give much more careful and thoughtful attention to the patient's 'persona', in both its individual and its social context. Our century has therefore witnessed the development of 'intimate personalisation' as well as 'social personalisation' in medical practice.

The chief evidence of the first has been the progressive introduction of psychotherapy into medical practice. Of course many doctors, perhaps the majority, do not yet use psycho-therapeutic techniques. Why is this? I believe there are two reasons: the time and patience that psychotherapy demands of both doctor and patient, and the customary discrepancy – at least in a good many European countries – between academically taught medicine and medicine as it is practised in the field. One proof of this, among many others, is the fact that future psychotherapists almost always have to learn their profession outside the Faculty of Medicine. But in spite of this, psychotherapy has become, since the years when Freud worked alone in the Berggasse, steadily more important to a doctor's practice and ideas.

The personalisation of medicine – 'the introduction of the subject', to use Weizsäcker's formula – has also been expressed in social terms. I am not referring here to the socialisation of medical practice that has taken place to some extent in every country; that I shall deal with shortly. At present I want to draw attention to the 'internal socialisation' that has clearly developed during the last few decades within the doctor-patient relationship and has affected several aspects of medical skill: in other words, to the fact that under subtle pressure from what is often called the 'spirit of the age' both diagnosis and treatment are becoming at the same time more personal and more social.

We find the same trend in the actual pattern of the treatment, especially of mental disorders *per se*. On one hand, the doctor knows how to adapt the individual's social position therapeutically – whether by group psychotherapy or psychodrama, collective rehabilitation, or use of hospital facilities. On the other hand, the treatment is aimed at reinstating the patient fully in his own social group – this is the significance of the great popularity of 'rehabilitation' at the present time. Moreover, the increasing technical complexity of modern medicine has led to the care of the sick being handed over to a medical team – which often includes non-medical technicians – at any rate in the important hospitals of large cities. Nothing could be more revealing, in this respect, than a quick glance at the historical development of the hospital. It began as an architectural and functional combination of infirmary and pharmacy; to this were successively added – not counting different therapeutic installations such as operating-theatres – a dissecting-room (seventeenth and eighteenth century), a chemical laboratory (first half of the nineteenth century) and a bacteriological laboratory (second half of the nineteenth century). Now, in the twentieth century, the hospital buildings are being 'socialised' and functionally planned for the benefit of the human beings who use them (departments of social welfare, social visitors, etc.), and the whole subject is itself being studied sociologically. The recent work of Hall, Schelsky, Biörck, Mitscherlich, Rohde, Caudill and others has given us a new understanding of the hospital as an institution: it is a community *sui generis,* whose sociological structure may either favour or retard therapy. As with the personality of the doctor, the hospital acts as its own medicine, sometimes beneficially and sometimes harmfully.

Before Pasteur, microbiology was not systematised;
after him, work on specific microbes as transmitters of disease
(Pasteur never claimed they were its cause) could go ahead.
The laboratory thus became part of the hospital
from the first half of the nineteenth century.

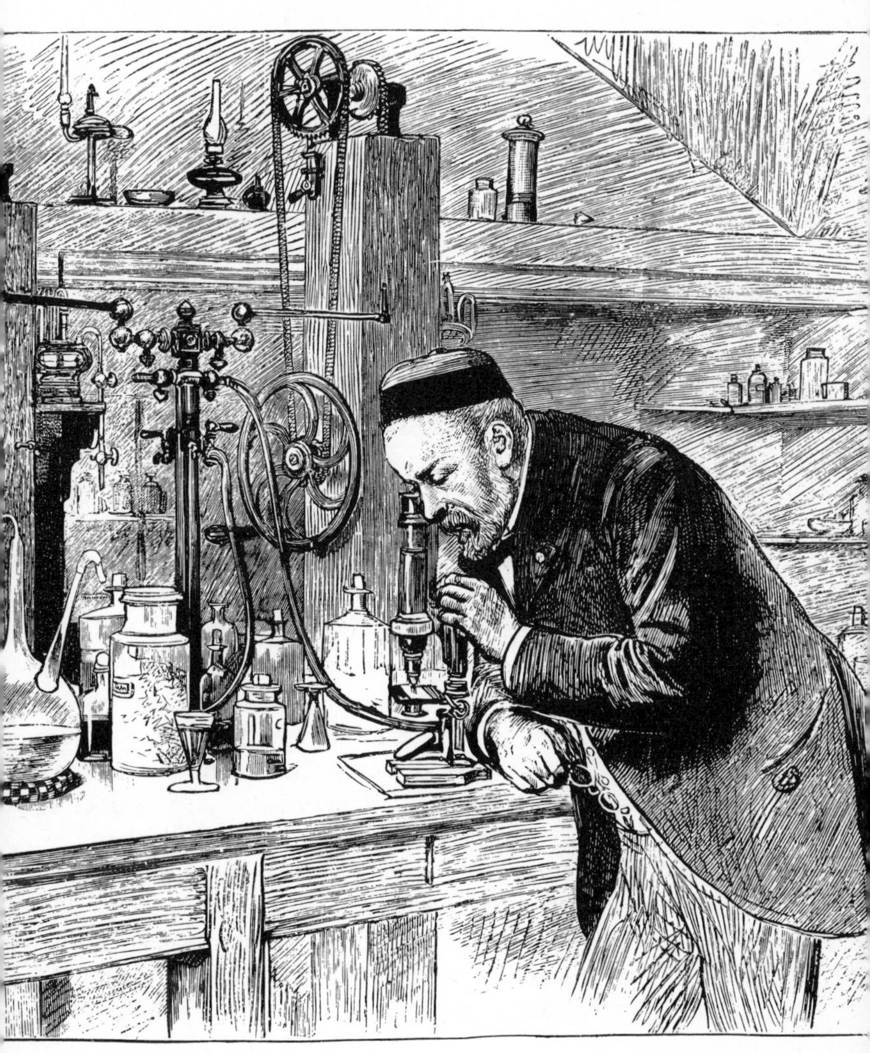

The social aspect

The reply given by the present century to the rebellion of the subject also has a social aspect, in the strongest and most commonly used sense of the expression. A strictly social principle – the suppression of the intolerable traditional difference between 'medicine for the rich' and 'medicine for the poor' – has made it obligatory to socialise medical assistance to a certain extent; this is the 'external socialisation' of medicine already referred to. Since Bismarck's law creating the *Krankenkassen* in Germany in 1883, to the National Health Insurance systems of Great Britain and Spain, and including the total socialisation of medical care in the Soviet Union and other socialist countries, there is hardly a civilised country which has not now made some fundamental change of one sort or another in the social structure by which technical assistance is given to the sick.

Cano Diaz has given the following pointful reasons explaining and justifying this partial or complete socialisation of medicine:

1 Modern medicine is both extremely effective and in very short supply. Diagnostic and therapeutic methods are at the same time very effective and very expensive. Again, doctors are much more frequently consulted than they used to be.

2 The sanitary conditions in which most of the population live, particularly the proletariat, are often deficient.

3 The general acceptance of the fact that man has a right to health. 'The enjoyment of the highest possible degree of health', says the WHO charter, 'is one of the fundamental

rights of every human being, regardless of race, religion, political ideology or economic and social status'.

4 The general modern tendency to socialise professions and skills.

5 The increasing intervention of the state in social life.

In my view there have been five chief manifestations of this decisive event:

1 The conscience of the man in the street of today – not merely that of social revolutionaries or persons of delicate moral sensibility – is violently opposed to discrimination in therapy on economic grounds. Such discrimination still exists to some extent, but a battle against it is going on all over the world.

2 The attitude of poor patients has radically changed. From the Middle Ages until the present century, hospital patients handed themselves over unconditionally to a medical service conceived of as charity where they were concerned. During the last decades, awareness that they have a radical and incontestable right to be looked after when they are ill has arisen and grown stronger among the working classes; and this has inevitably emphasised the contractual character of the medical relationship.

3 Medical care of the impoverished sick was once normally limited to cases of serious organic illness. Today every invalid feels he has the right to seek professional help for slight illnesses, even when they are functional or neurotic.

4 Until the twentieth century, illness in a poor person was, quite simply a disaster. For the last few years, although it is still considered a slight or serious misfortune, illness has come

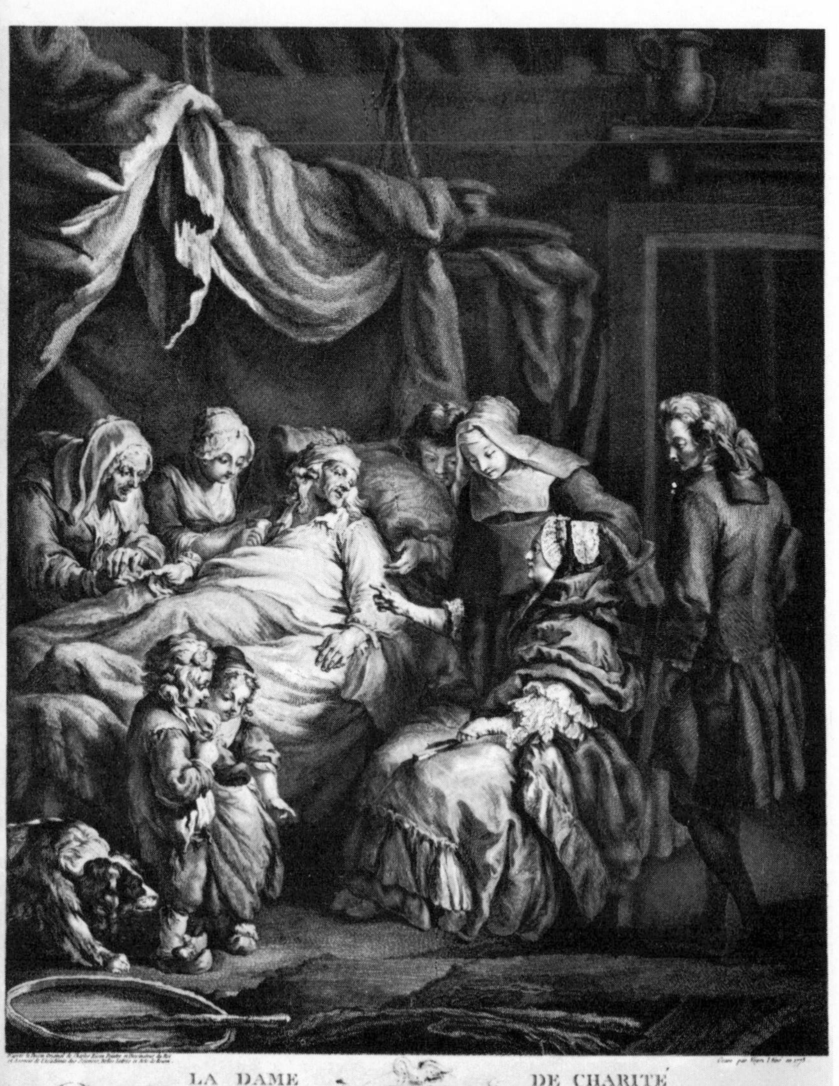
LA DAME DE CHARITÉ
Dédiée à Madame Marie Charlotte de Bethune Comtesse de Tessé Douairière, Grande d'Espagne de la 1re Classe. &c.a
A Paris chez Le Bas et Aveline Md.s d'Estampes rue St
Par Ses très humbles et très Obéissants

Two illustrations of medical institutions in the eighteenth century. *Left* La Dame de Charité, by Charles Eisen. Court ladies would give time to visiting the sick, generally at the many charity hospitals. *Below* The Naples Health Office. This centre for quarantine enforcement in the port was an early instance of preventive medicine in public health.

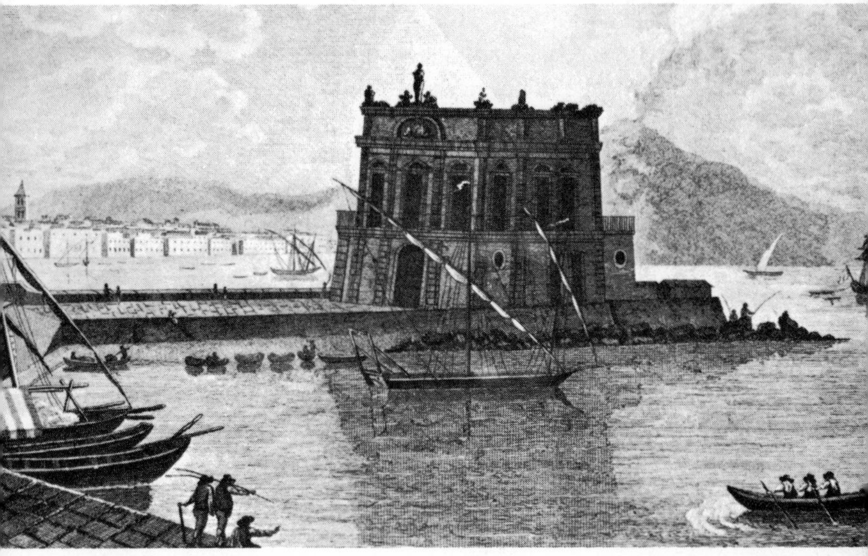

to be considered as a source of extra-medical privileges: a poor invalid is entirely justified in thinking that his sufferings entitle him to some personal and social compensation.

5 Medical care of the impoverished sick has had to be organised collectively, and subjected to some form of bureaucracy. Doctors are now officials as well as clinicians.

It is plain that in our century medical care has been socialised on strictly social principles 'from without'. A crucial time has begun for private practice and traditional hospital treatment. The old charity hospital is vanishing in every country. Except in the most economically independent or politically important social strata, the sick are usually taken care of by some form of health insurance. The medical relationship of today is most commonly established within this framework. What effect has this had upon it?

Before answering the question, we must glance rapidly at another feature of present-day life and medicine: the social habit that Luis Alberti has called the 'autonomy of techniques'. Most of man's vital needs can in fact be satisfied today by objects that are either mass-produced or whose manufacture needs no special skill. One has only to think of the contrast between getting a chemist to make up a special prescription a hundred years ago, and buying a bottle of aspirins in any pharmacy today. It is hardly an exaggeration to speak of 'medication without doctors or chemists'. Analgesics, hypnotics and tranquilisers, antibiotics and laxatives – thousands of pharmaceutical products in fact – can be obtained today without any visible intervention of the technician who prepared them or the slightest participation of those who understand their purpose and ought to prescribe them. In fact, medication has become a social benefit within reach of anyone who can afford it.

Personalisation and socialisation of medicine, complexity and increasing autonomy of the techniques of diagnosis and therapy – these are the internal and external conditions that determine the relation between doctor and patient today. However, the final form it has taken is different in the two great politico-social spheres which make up the western world of today – the 'capitalist' and 'socialist' societies.

The problem of socialised medicine

Whether complete or partial, the socialisation of the care of the sick is without any doubt at all the most important feature of present-day medicine. To conclude our investigation of the relation between doctor and patient in the world of today, we will take a synoptic view of the possibilities that have been opened up, and the problems raised, by this socialisation of medicine. Let us simplify matters by admitting that the technical training of doctors and the functional capacity of the health services (administrative system, methods of diagnosis, and therapy, etc.), are adequate. What will be, and what could be, the medical relation within this organisation? If we contemplate at the same time the empirical reality (what really happens), the possible reality (what might happen if the available facilities were properly used), and the ideal reality (what would happen under the best possible conditions), we are faced with three different sorts of problem:

1 Problems of an affective sort. Unless the patient is completely free to choose his doctor, can a true 'medical philia' possibly be established between them? Faithful consideration of this question obliges us to break up the question into others that are simpler and more precise.

Is the patient's confidence in his doctor, though always advantageous, an absolutely necessary condition for a correct diagnosis and effective treatment? If the diagnostic and therapeutic methods in use are objectively effective and if the patient is psychologically sane and healthy, the reply must be negative. A lobar pneumonia or a fractured bone can be very correctly diagnosed and very effectively treated without this confidence ever having been established. Therapeutic remedies are effective principally by reason of their intrinsic qualities, and although the patient's lack of confidence may diminish the favourable action, it will not prevent penicillin destroying the pneumococci, or the formation of callus round the fracture.

Is free choice of his doctor necessary to the patient's confidence in him? In the last analysis, no. A doctor whom the patient has not chosen can almost always, if he really tries, gain his confidence. Two simple conditions, technical adequacy and goodwill, will usually suffice. And it is his duty to succeed if he can.

Have patients ever really been completely free to choose their doctor? The truth is that this privilege has only been available on the whole to those in positions of power. A hospital patient used to be attended by the head of the department to which he was sent, or perhaps by some subordinate doctor whose name he did not even know; and it was the same, *mutatis mutandis,* with country patients. Let us be honest: below a certain economic level, the patient's freedom to choose his doctor has been in the immense majority of cases a purely nominal right.

I want to make myself perfectly clear. I am in no way trying to say that it is not better for a patient to be free to choose his doctor than to lack that freedom. Some power of choice is both possible and advantageous, as is shown by the health insurance systems of France, Germany and Great Britain, among others. Nevertheless, I think the problem should be fairly stated. Here is my thesis: perfect clinical practice necessitates the patient's confidence in his doctor, and this is more easily achieved when the principle of free choice prevails; but this does not prevent medical care of a very acceptable quality being provided even without freedom of choice, given the conditions I have mentioned.

2 Problems of a technico-economic nature. Although the training of doctors may be adequate, without competent organisation and without money – without a great deal of money – socialised medicine can never be fairly distributed and efficient. Under its superficial organisation, the old contrast between 'medicine for the rich' and 'medicine for the poor' will persist almost intact.

I am not referring only to the high cost of modern installations and the enormous range of therapeutic equipment; I am also thinking of the fees of the innumerable doctors employed in the service. Unless doctors are guaranteed a decent standard of living, is it legitimate to expect the goodwill from them to which I have so often referred? Unless there is a sufficiency of general practitioners and specialists to provide those in their care with modern techniques of healing, how can an insured person be properly treated? Let us consider for a moment how many kinds of doctors are required by any health organisation that hopes to provide a satisfactory service – general practitioners, specialists in hospital or public health work, biochemists, pathologists, bacteriologists, radiologists, physiotherapists, psychiatrists, social workers and so forth – and then let us remember what has already been said about the time devoted to each patient. As Napoleon said of war, socialised medicine requires, besides technique and organisation, 'money, money, and money'.

3 Problems of a moral order. Without a thriving 'social morality' – a morality directed at ends affecting society rather than the next man – can socialised medical care be satisfactory? Such ethical considerations are equally relevant to patient, doctor and administrative official.

An insured person is usually conscious of a twofold right – to medical care that is humanly and technically satisfactory, and to indemnification. From the point of view of social justice, both are morally unquestionable. But except for the counter-balancing obligations corresponding to them, may they not be a source of difficulties and conflicts in the medical relation? Consciousness of a right to medical care should be accompanied by a determined and disciplined desire to get well; otherwise – Parsons' sociological scheme is relevant here – it will become morally and socially corrupt. The right to indemnification must be objectively and subjectively based on an obligation not to treat it as plunder or profit. Malingering is the most flagrant example of lack of moral sense on the patient's part, but not the only one: there also exists the wide, but clinically, morally and socially undefined field surrounding the compensation neuroses, or neuroses of exemption, by which a great many individuals half-way between health and illness make use of not entirely unconscious mechanisms as a means to avoid obligations or to achieve financial gain.

Moral danger for the patient lies in consciously abusing one

A right to medical care. The penicillin injection programme supported by WHO and UNICEF visits one of Indonesia's 3,000 islands in the struggle against yaws. More sophisticated, the health insurance of richer countries compels a closer definition of this 'right' and how it is to be secured by doctors and patients.

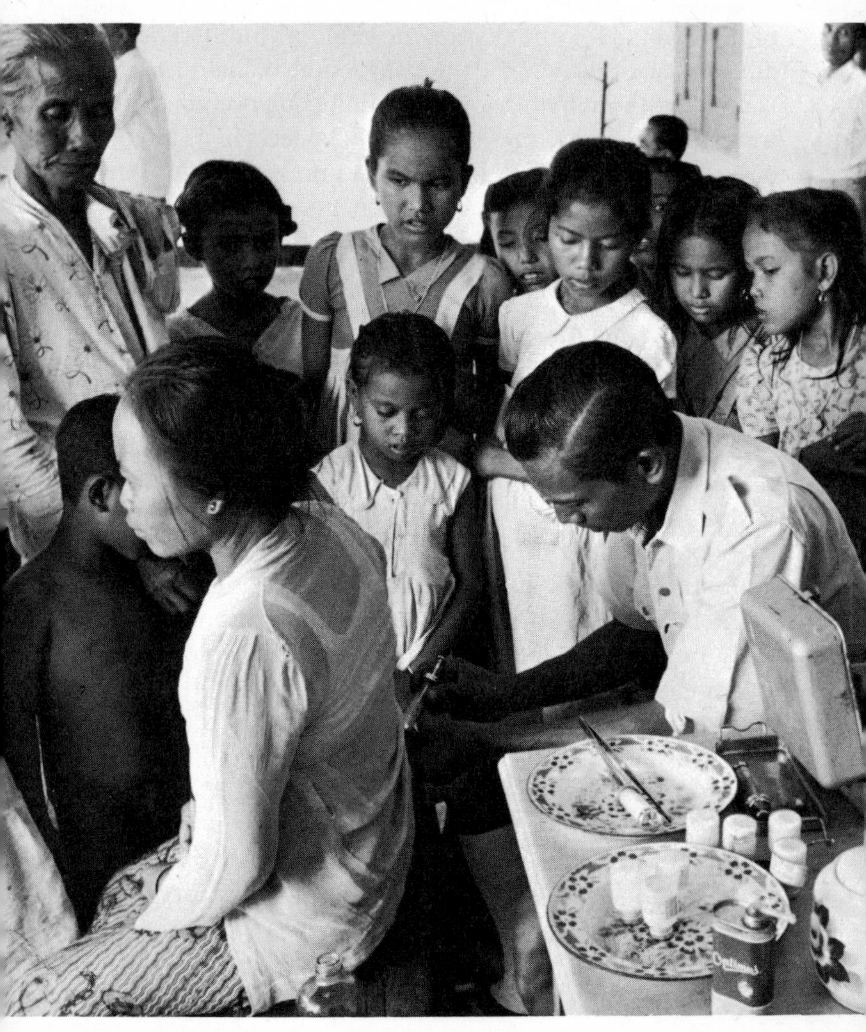

of his rights; for the doctor, in habitual indifference to his duties – in other words, the conversion of his practice into routine. Although his technical training may be adequate, can we exonerate a doctor who, because he feels he is an 'official' or – even worse – because he thinks no zeal on his part can increase his earnings, only gives his patient perfunctory treatment? Morally and emotionally, the doctor's situation with regard to health insurance schemes is not usually a happy one. He has to look after too many patients. He knows that he is to a certain extent responsible for the sanitary conditions of the society to which he belongs. The efforts he must make to keep his medical knowledge up to date and carry out his clinical tasks properly are not usually recognised. Because he must write medical certificates for his patients, he has to act as a judge, faced by all the delicate emotional and moral problems that such decisions so often involve. If in addition to all this his remuneration is too low, must he not often be tempted to give perfunctory or routine treatment? Only one way lies ahead of him: that indicated by the old Latin maxim *hic Rhodus, hic salta*.

An administrative official must, in fact, resist the temptation of confusing 'function' with 'ownership'. The chief aim of the health service is to give medical aid, and the protagonists in this are patient and doctor. There are few more disturbing features of socialised medical care than this corrupt conversion of the administrators of a public service into its proprietors.

Verdict on socialised medicine

Perhaps we are now in a position to make a critical appraisal of this decisive development in medicine, from the point of view of the relation between doctor and patient.

It must first be said that, taken as a whole, the socialisation of medical care is a just, irreversible and progressive historical event. The famous theological argument of Duns Scotus could well be applied to it: *potuit, decuit, ergo fecit.* But the historical necessity and indubitable justice of this event should not make the manner of its technical and social realisation immune to criticism. On the contrary. Since all health insurance organisations from Bismarck's *Krankenkassen* to the systems in force today in Great Britain, the Soviet Union or elsewhere are merely tentative approaches towards some less unsatisfactory medical service, the easiest – but not the least serious – form of injustice would be to take a negative attitude towards their revision. The world has never been static, but seldom has it so fully deserved to be called a 'changing world' as it does today.

The doctor-patient relationship in socialised medicine of the present day is very far from satisfactory. Very briefly, these are the reasons:

1 The short time devoted to each patient by his doctor. If it is impossible to give full attention to the diagnosis and therapy of each of his patients, how can real medical philia be formed in his practice?

2 The lack of incentives, not only economic ones, usually offered to the doctor by the health service.

3 In quite a number of cases the organisation of services is unsatisfactory, because of restrictions in the choice of a doctor and in the range of diagnostic and therapeutic expedients the doctor is allowed to prescribe.
4 The social education of the doctor is often inadequate. Education in many countries does not sufficiently arouse a co-operative moral sense in the individual. Also the Medical Faculties are often blind or myopic in their attitude to the extremely varied problems presented at the present time by the relation between illness and society.
5 The education of the patient as a citizen and member of society is often just as defective. He is usually far more conscious of his rights as an invalid than of his duties to society – which is not an abstract entity but a collection of human beings, only a few of them known to him. No doubt he cannot be expected to abandon 'competitive morality' (personal gain either in the form of money or fame will always be a powerful incentive to the sons of Adam); but competition of an emulative or fratricidal sort is only permissible when subordinated to 'co-operative morality'.

To this list of defects should be added another list – of reforms to be aimed at. Different countries will adopt very different rhythms in the steady improvement and revision required by socialised medical care. Where this rhythm is slow and ineffectual, should a doctor take the line: 'Since they don't listen to what I say, I can't do my duty properly'? If the health and lives of other men were not at stake perhaps he should; but its aims are such that the medical profession always exacts complete submission from the practitioner.

Herein lies the servitude of the medical profession but also its moral greatness. And it is the main reason why socialised medicine all over the world is a developing enterprise.

7 Conclusion

This investigation of the relation between doctor and patient in the history of the West and the world of today leads us to confirm, I think, the brilliant perspicacity of the ancient Greeks when they called this relation *philia,* or 'friendship'. When this bond is truly what it should be, it produces a special form of friendly communication – 'medical philia'. It does not matter whether this understanding takes place between minds of ancient Greeks, of Christians, or of modern and secularised men. Insofar as man is a part of nature, and health an aspect of this nature and therefore a natural and objective good, the medical relation develops into comradeship, or association for the purpose of securing this good by technical means. Insofar as man is an individual and his illness a state affecting his personality, the medical relation ought to be more than mere comradeship – in fact it should be friendship. All dogma apart, a good doctor has always been a friend to his patient, to all his patients. And the patient for his part tries to surmount every psychological and social barrier and be a real friend to his doctor, and often succeeds. Few invalids who are properly looked after will fail to endorse the words of Seneca which introduce this book.

But if this ideal medical philia is to be achieved, a whole series of obstacles belonging to every historical and social situation must be overcome. Some have cropped up monotonously since the days of ancient Greece: lack of skill, excessive desire for money, inhuman dogmatism, carelessness, laziness or bad temper on the doctor's part; fickleness, intemperance or extreme egotism on the patient's. Others are peculiar to the environment in which the medical relation is formed: superstitious awe of Asclepius in ancient Greece; pseudo-Christian superstition and the 'ordalian' outlook of the Middle Ages; exaggerated awareness of rights, and contentiousness in our time. But such obstacles seldom prevent a technically well-trained and morally admirable doctor from forming a satisfactory medical relation with his patients, and therefore a friendly one.

Will technical progress perhaps bring with it a form of medicine in which a direct relation between doctor and patient plays no part? Will a doctor become for the morbid disorders of the human organism what an engineer is for a breakdown in a motor? I do not think so. I believe there will always be disease because the disposition to disease, and disease itself are constituent parts of the human condition; and I am sure that when he is ill man will almost always call upon his doctor for technical help. While there are men there will be diseases and doctors.

With seriousness tinged with humour – or with humour streaked with seriousness, whichever you prefer – the biologist Jean Rostand imagined what an experimentally produced specimen of *homo biologicus* would say about himself: 'I am the product of carefully selected semen irradiated with neutrons; my sex was predetermined and I was incubated by a mother who was not mine; I was given injections of hormones and DNA during gestation, and subjected to activation of the cortex; after I was born my intellectual development was stimulated by several grafts; at the present time I am having annual treatments to keep my mind at its best and my instincts in full vigour. I cannot complain of my body, my sex or my life. But what am I, in fact?' Let us complete Jean Rostand's joke, and reply to *homo biologicus*: 'You are a being capable of falling ill, and who will fall ill one of these days. And then, in the very depths of your being, you will feel a need to be cared for and helped by a man with special technical knowledge, who is prepared to treat you as a friend. In short, a good doctor.'

Notes

1 Some may object that the word *philanthrôpia* was invented after almost all the *Corpus Hippocraticum* was written. This is true, as it is also true that the *Praecepta*, the only Hippocratic writing in which this word appears, was a very late work (U. Fleischer). But a careful study of the Hippocratic writings leads to the conclusion that Hippocrates and his direct and indirect followers were 'philanthropists' *avant la lettre*.

2 See my book *La curación por la palabra en la Antigüedad clásica* (Madrid 1958).

3 The formally Christian version of this behaviour – and therefore of neighbourliness – is based on three evangelical precepts: (1) Thou shalt love thy neighbour as thyself. (2) Love thy neighbour as if he were Jesus Christ. (3) Love thy neighbour as if thou thyself were Jesus Christ. The texts in which these precepts appear are well known.

4 This treatise by Archimateus is an amplification of an anonymous work called *De adventu medici ad aegrotum*.

5 Further details in my book *La historia clinica* (2nd edition, Barcelona 1961).

6 This significant phrase is quoted by G. von Bergmann in his *Funktionelle Pathologie* (Berlin 1932).

7 For details see García-Sabell *Antropología del hombre gallego enfermo* (Vigo, Salicia 1964).

8 See Pittenger, Danehy and Kockett *The First Five Minutes. A Sample of Microscopic Interview Analysis* (Paul Martineau 1961).

9 See J. A. L. Singh and R. L. Zingg *The Wolf-children and feral-man* (New York 1942).

10 It is hardly necessary to say that the situation becomes even more subtle and complex in the case of neurotics in the strict sense; see my book *La relación médico-enfermo* (Madrid 1964).

11 This brief summary by no means exhausts Parsons' sociological analysis of the medical profession. The doctor's role, like others, is subjected to 'pattern variables', which are five in his case. Social considerations in fact force the doctor to choose (1) between emotion and affective neutrality; (2) between universalism and particularism; (3) between orientation towards collectivity and self-orientation; (4) between considering the patient's personal circumstances or exclusively considering his social efficiency; (5) between a functionally diffuse or a functionally specific orientation. In a modern civilised society, a doctor must be affectively neutral, orientated towards collectivity, prefer universalism, put social efficiency first, and act in a strictly specific manner. Other factors could be added to this analysis.

Bibliography

1 Classical Greece

Ever since the first philological study of the *Corpus Hippocraticum* by Fredrich (*Hippokratische Untersuchungen*, Berlin, 1899), the bibliography of Hippocratic medicine has steadily increased. A complete summary of this bibliography would be out of place here. Readers interested in the subject can consult:
L. Edelstein, 'Hippokrates', *Realencyclopädie* of Pauly-Wissowa, Supplement-Band VI, Stuttgart, 1935; H. Diller, *Wanderarzt und Aitiologie*, Leipzig, 1934 and *Stand und Aufgaben der Hippokratesforschung*, Mainz, 1959; K. Deichgräber, *Die Epidemien und das Corpus Hippocraticum*, Berlin, 1934 and 'Die Stellung des griechischen Arztes zur Natur', *Die Antike* XV, Berlin, 1939; W. Jaeger, *Paideia*, vol. III; W. Nestle, 'Hippocratica', *Griechische Studien*, Stuttgart, 1948; W. Jones, *Philosophy and Medicine in Ancient Greece*, Baltimore, 1946; P. Lain-Entralgo, *La curación por la palabra en la Antigüedad clásica,* Madrid, 1958; M. Martiny, *Hippocrate et la médecine*, Paris, 1964. There are important papers also by H. W. Miller in *Transactions and Proceedings of the American Philological Association*, 1953 et seq. In *Der Arzt im Altertum*, Munich, 3rd ed., 1962, W. Müri has published an excellent selection of classical medical texts.

Textual references to the *Corpus Hippocraticum* are always based on Littré's edition; the number of the volume is given in Roman and the page number in Arabic figures.

On the Greek notion of friendship, apart from such early works as E. Curtius, *Althertum und Gegenwart*, 4th ed., Berlin, 1892, and L. Dugas, *L'amitié antique*, Paris, 1894, and other studies, see: J. J. Verbrugh, *Über platonische Freundschaft*, Diss. Zürich, 1931; P. Kienzl, *Die Theorie der Liebe und Freundschaft bei Platon*, Diss. Wien, 1941; E. Hoffmann, 'Aristoteles Philosophie der Freundschaft', *Platonismus und christliche Philosophie*, Zürich and Stuttgart, 1960.

The social and economic structure of the Greek *polis* has been recently studied in *Sozialökonomische Verhältnisse im Alten Orient und im Klassischen Altertums*, Berlin, 1961.

The ethics of the Hippocratic Asclepiads have been described and criticised by G. Weiss, 'Die ethischen Anschauungen im Corpus Hippocraticum', *Archiv für Geschichte der Medizin* IV, 1910, 235-62; L. Edelstein, *The Hippocratic Oath*, Baltimore, 1946; K. Deichgräber, *Der Hippokratische Eid*, Stuttgart, 1955; F. Büchner, *Der Eid des Hippokrates*, Freiburg, i. Br., 1945.

2 The Middle Ages

To amplify the contents of this chapter, the reader may consult general histories of medicine, as well as my book *La Relación médico-enfermo*, Madrid, 1964, already mentioned, and the following books and articles:

A. Ruiz Moreno, *La medicina en la legislación medioeval española*, Buenos Aires, 1946; K. Sudhoff, 'Eine Verteidigung der Heilkunde aus der Zeiten der Mönchsmedizin', *Archiv für Geschichte der Medizin* VII, 1913, 223-37; Coluccio Salutati, *De nobilitate legum et medicinae*, ed. E. Garin, Florence, 1947; E. Seidler, 'Die Heilkunde des ausgehenden Mittelalters in Paris', *Beihefte des Sudhoffs Archivs*, Wiesbaden, 1967.

3 The nineteenth century

Nineteenth-century literature often reflects the relationship between doctor and patient during that period. See *La relation médecin-malade dans l'oeuvre romanesque de Flaubert et de Proust*, Thèse de

Paris, 1962; L. Garcia Ballester, 'El testimonio de la sociedad española en el siglo XIX acerca del médico y su actividad', *Medicina y sociedad en la España del siglo* XIX, Madrid, 1964.

For a more detailed picture of the social aspects of the medical relationship during this century, the following books and articles may be consulted:

C. Turner Thackrah, *The Effects of Principal Arts, Trades, and Professions and of Civic States and Habits of Living, on Health and Longevity*, London, 1831; E. Chadwick, *Report on the Sanitary Conditions of the Labouring Population of Great Britain*, London, 1842; H. E. Sigerist, *Medicine and Human Welfare*, New Haven, 1941 and *Civilización y enfermedad*, Mexico, 1964; R. Pierreville, *L'inegalité humaine devant la mort et la maladie,* Paris, 1936; M. Delabroise, *Louis René Villermé*, Paris, 1939; C. Fecan, *Le rapport Villermé,* Thèse de Paris, 1962; Rollo H. Britten, *Public Health Reports,* vol. 49, 1934; G. St J. Perrott and S. D. Collins, *Public Health Reports*, vol. 50, 1935; J. M. López Piñero, 'El testimonio de los médicos españoles del siglo XIX acerca de la sociedad de su tiempo: el proletariado industrial', in *Medicina y sociedad en la España del siglo* XIX, Madrid, 1964. The sociological aspects of hysteria in the Salpêtrière have been studied by G. Bally in *Einführung in die Psychoanalyse Sigmund Freuds*, Hamburg, 1961.

4 The basis of the relationship

I refer the reader again to my books *La relación médico-enfermo* and *Teoría y realidad del Otro*.

Here is a selective bibliography of works dealing with the subjects referred to in this chapter:

E. Koos, 'Metropolis. What city people think of their medical services', *Am. J. Public Health,* 45, 1955, 1551-7; R. H. Blum,

Hospitals and Patient Dissatisfaction, Calif. Med. Assoc. 1958 and *Physician-Patient Relationship, Survey and Action,* Calif. Med. Assoc. 1956.

On the feeling of being ill:
Th. von Uexküll, 'Das Problem der Befindenweisen', *Psyche* v, 1951, 401-32; H.Plügge, 'Die Phänomenologie des Leiberlebens', in *Rencontre-Encounter-Begegnung*, Utrecht-Antwerpen, 1957; J.de Ajuriaguerra, 'Le corps comme relation', *Rev. Suisse de Psychologie pure et appliquée,* XXI, 1962, 137-57; H.Häfner, 'Psychosomatische Medizin und Leibphänomenologie', *Werden und Handeln*, Stuttgart, 1963; J.J.López Ibor, 'Anatomía del intracuerpo', *Atlántida* I, 1963, 5-12; and of course E. Kretschmer's classic *Medizinische Psychologie.* The social aspects of the feeling of being ill have been studied by E.Ackerknecht, 'The role of medical history in medical education', *Bull. Hist. Med.* 21, 1947, 135-45; J.C.Lawson, *Modern Greek Folklore and Ancient Greek Religion*, London, 1910; E.L.Koos, *The Health of Regionville*, New York, 1954; M.Zborowski, 'Cultural components in response to pain', *J. Social Issues* 8, 1952, 16-30. A more extensive bibliography on the subject is found in M. Pflanz, *Sozialer Wandel und Krankheit,* Stuttgart, 1962; R.H.Blum, J.Sadusk and R.Waterson, *The Management of the Doctor-Patient-Relationship,* New York-Toronto-London, 1960; and others. For the psychology of medical consultation, see the article by W. Schulte, 'Der nächste Patient', *Werden und Handeln*, Stuttgart, 1963.

5 The structure of the relationship

On the psychology of looking, see my book *Teoría y realidad del Otro*, and the bibliography it contains. I have gone more fully into the theory of clinical anamnesis indicated here in my books *La historia clínica* and *La relación médico-enfermo*. I refer the reader also to R. E. Pittenger, J. Danehy and Ch. F. Kockett, *The First Five Minutes. A Sample of Microscopic Interview Analysis,* Paul Martineau, 1961, and to J. Rof Carballo, 'La teoría de la comunicación en la medicina contemporánea', *Anales de la Sociedad de Ciencias Médicas de Las Palmas*, I, 1962. The role of cybernetics in clinical diagnosis has been systematically studied by F. Paycha, *Cybernétique et consultation*, Paris, 1963, among others, and the symbolical character of exploratory instruments by J. P. Valabrega, *La relation thérapeutique*, Paris, 1962.

The psychoanalytical doctrine of the transference has been fully documented in M. Steinbach, 'Die Übertragung. Geschichte und Entwicklung einer Theorie', *Psyche* VII, 1953, 6-25, and D. Lagache, 'La doctrine freudienne et la théorie du Transfert', *Acta Psychosom. et Orthopaed.,* 2, 1954. On the counter-transference, see C. A. Seguín, *Amor y psicoterapia,* Buenos Aires, 1963, and R. A. Spitz, 'Übertragung und Gegenübertragung' *Psyche* X, 1956-7, 63-81. *The Doctor, his Patient and the Illness,* M. Balint, New York, 1957, is almost a classic on this subject. See also: R. M. Magraw, *Ferment in Medicine,* Philadelphia and London, 1966.

For an introduction to a more detailed study of the social aspects of the medical relationship, see the book by M. Pflanz mentioned above, and also Talcott Parsons, *The Social System,* Glencoe, 1951, a special number of the *Kölner Zeitschrift für Soziologie*, 1958, devoted to the sociological problems of medicine, as well as the essays collected in *Der Kranke in der modernen Gesellschaft*, Cologne -Berlin, 1967. But in the true medical relationship there exists an 'interpersonal' bond, within the social framework. For references to this theme see P. Christian, *Das Personvertändnis im modernen medizinischen Denken*, Tübingen, 1952; A. Maeder, *Der Psychotherapeut als Partner,* Zürich, 1957; J. Rof Carballo, *Urdimbre afectiva y enfermedad,* Barcelona-Madrid, 1961.

6 The relationship today

On the gradual 'internal socialisation' of the medical relationship during the twentieth century, see:
V. von Weizsäcker, *Soziale Krankheit und soziale Gesundung*, Leipzig, 1930; H. Schelsky, 'Die Soziologie des Krankenhauses im Rahmen einer Soziologie der Medizin', *Krankenhausarzt* 31, 1958, 169; W. Sottstaedt and others, 'Sociology, psychology and metabolic observations in the community of a metabolic ward', *Am. J. Med.* 25, 1958, 248, and 'Prestige and social interactions on a metabolic ward', *Psychosomat. Med.* 21, 1959, 131; W. Caudill, *The Psychiatric Hospital as a Small Society*, Cambridge, Mass., 1959; J. Rof Carballo, 'Idea del hombre, medicina y sociedad', *Rev. de la Universidad de Madrid* x, 1961, 155-206.

A panoramic view of the 'external socialisation' of this relationship – present-day socialisation of medical aid – has been given by P. Cano Díaz in 'El Seguro de Enfermedad en el mundo occidental', *Rev. de la Universidad de Madrid* x, 1961, 207–44. For information concerning medical services in the Soviet Union, see the bibliography included in the text.

Acknowledgments

Acknowledgment – further to any made in the captions – is due to the following for illustrations (the number refers to the page on which the illustration appears): 50, 80, 92, 117, 133, 161, 164, 214-5, 227 The Wellcome Trustees; 55, 68-9 Bibliothèque Nationale, Paris; 58 Österreichische National-Bibliothek; 63, 69, 72-3, 76, 85, 89, 93, 109, 110, 115, 129, 142, 230 British Museum; 84, 96 Fitzwilliam Museum, Cambridge; 104, 220 St Bartholomew's Hospital; 116 Librairie Hachette; 136, 139, 184 Mrs Katharine Jones and The Hogarth Press; 144 Mr Ernst Freud; 153, 168-9, 189 Radio Times Hulton Picture Library; 174, 218 (Paul Almasy), 237 (H. Page) World Health Organisation; 200-1 The Mansell Collection.

Index

World University Library

Some titles already published

001 **Eye and Brain**
R. L. Gregory, *Edinburgh*

002 **The Economics of Underdeveloped Countries**
Jagdish Bhagwati, *MIT*

003 **The Left in Europe since 1789**
David Caute, *London*

004 **The World Cities**
Peter Hall, *Reading*

005 **Chinese Communism**
Robert North, *Stanford*

006 **The Emergence of Greek Democracy**
W. G. Forrest, *Oxford*

009 **Palaeolithic Cave Art**
P. J. Ucko and A. Rosenfeld, *London*

011 **Russian Writers and Society 1825-1904**
Ronald Hingley, *Oxford*

013 **Education in the Modern World**
John Vaizey, *London*

014 **The Rise of Toleration**
Henry Kamen, *Warwick*

015 **Art Nouveau**
S. Tschudi Madsen, *Oslo*

017 **Decisive Forces in World Economics**
J. L. Sampedro, *Madrid*

018 **Development Planning**
Jan Tinbergen, *Rotterdam*

019 **Human Communication**
J. L. Aranguren, *Madrid*

021 **The Rise of the Working Class**
Jürgen Kuczynski, *Berlin*

022 **The Science of Decision-making**
A. Kaufmann, *Paris*

023 **Chinese Medicine**
P. Huard and M. Wong, *Paris*

024 **Muhammad and the Conquests of Islam**
Francesco Gabrieli, *Rome*

025 **Humanism in the Renaissance**
S. Dresden, *Leyden*

028 **The Age of the Dinosaurs**
Björn Kurtén, *Helsingfors*

029 **Mimicry in Plants and Animals**
Wolfgang Wickler, *Seewiesen*

030 **The Old Stone Age**
François Bordes, *Bordeaux*

032 **The Civilisation of Charlemagne**
Jacques Boussard, *Poitiers*

034 **The Dutch Republic**
C. H. Wilson, *Cambridge*

038 **The Tasks of Childhood**
Philippe Muller, *Neuchâtel*

039 **Twentieth Century Music**
H. H. Stuckenschmidt, *Berlin*

041 **Witchcraft**
Lucy Mair, *London*

042 **Population and History**
E. A. Wrigley, *Cambridge*

043 **Satire**
Matthew Hodgart, *Sussex*

044 **Christian Monasticism**
David Knowles, *Cambridge*

045 **The Italian City-Republics**
Daniel Waley, *London*